THE JUICE MASTER DIET

JASON VALE

7 lbs IN 7 DAYS

New and Updated Edition

Other books by the Juice Master

THE JUICE MASTER DIET

JASON VALE

7 lbs IN 7 DAYS

'The Juice Programme works! And if it can work for me I believe it can work for anyone.'

Jordan

HarperCollins*Publishers*
77–85 Fulham Palace Road,
Hammersmith, London W6 8JB

www.harpercollins.co.uk

H A R P E R ™
thorsons

and HarperThorsons are trademarks of
HarperCollins*Publishers* Ltd

First published as *7lbs in 7 Days Super Juice Diet* by HarperThorsons 2006
This edition published 2012

3

A catalogue record of this book is
available from the British Library

ISBN 978-0-00-743618-7

Printed and bound in Great Britain by
Clays Ltd, St Ives plc

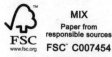

MIX
Paper from
responsible sources
FSC
www.fsc.org   FSC™ C007454

FSC™ is a non-profit international organisation established to promote
the responsible management of the world's forests. Products carrying the
FSC label are independently certified to assure consumers that they come
from forests that are managed to meet the social, economic and
ecological needs of present and future generations,
and other controlled sources.

Find out more about HarperCollins and the environment at
www.harpercollins.co.uk/green

Contents

THE JUICE MASTER DIET

JASON VALE

7lbs IN 7 DAYS

Introduction:
Juicing Changed My Life!

Juicing has changed my life beyond all recognition. I know it's a cliché when people say this or that changed their life, but I can say with total confidence that without juicing my life would be radically different to what it is today.

Before I got into juicing I used to smoke 40–60 cigarettes a day; I liked my drink (as they say); I was more than partial to the odd bit of junk(ie) food, and, as a result, I was also fat. On top of that I had severe asthma to the point where I had to use both the blue and brown inhalers and was having 10–16 puffs a day on them. I also developed eczema, mild acne, bad hay fever, and very, very severe psoriasis. In short, I wasn't exactly in the best of health and my energy levels were often right through the floor.

I am now in the fortunate position of being free from smoking, drinking and junk food. My asthma has vanished, my eczema and acne have gone, my psoriasis has cleared by over 90% and I am no longer overweight. In fact, on the health front I'm one happy camper!

I am now also lucky to be able to help people who find themselves in a similar position to the one I was in. Since the launch of my first book, *Slim for Life: Freedom from the Food Trap*, I have been blessed with tens of thousands of letters and e-mails from all over the world from people who have made incredible changes to their health and lives.

My previous book, *Turbo-Charge Your Life in 14 Days* exceeded all expectations when it reached number three in one of the best-seller charts (Harry Potter took the first two spots). It was written about in virtually every magazine as well as being discussed on TV and radio to the extent that several radio presenters followed the programme themselves and reported on their progress to the listeners.

The success of that book led to some of the most amazing letters about life-changing experiences I have ever had: people who not only lost an amazing amount of weight, but more importantly, whose lives had changed for good – not just for the two weeks. They had set out to do a quick 14-day plan to lose some weight and get a little healthier, only to find that their eating habits and lifestyle changed for good.

This was exactly what I had in mind with this programme, but the impacct this book has had throughout the world has taken everyone by surprise. It hit the number one slot and even knocked the *Da Vinci Code* off the top spot on one of the book charts. It has been translated into many languages and it was even reported that Sarah

Jessica Parker, Drew Barrymore and Jennifer Aniston have all done, what is now being called – The Juice Diet. I have no idea if they actually did the plan, but many celebrities have known about the weight-loss and health power of freshly extracted juice for years. The Super Juice Diet has been talked about on television and radio in many parts of the world and even many in the medical profession now recommend the programme. You won't believe how good you will look and feel in such a short space of time. I realize you should under-sell and over deliver, but there are now over one million copies of the book, DVD and now an app in homes throughout the world and I have read and seen the truly breathtaking results. This is why I have 100 per cent confidence in the programme, both as a weight loss tool and a health tool.

Diets Don't Work – **Do They?**

I realize that the subtitle of this book – *7lbs in 7 days* – may have lured many people into looking for some kind of 'quick fix', but I know that if you read the book and follow all of the instructions, it will be a catalyst to a *lifelong* change.

I have already been rapped for using the word 'diet' on the front cover of this book, but that's the publisher – not me! I did argue my case over and over again: after all, the first chapter in *Slim for Life* is all about why diets don't work, but here I am with a book that contains a title with the word 'diet' in it. I suppose that in order to get your message to the people who need it most you sometimes have to compromise along the way, and the title of this book is one of those compromises.

Having said that, after thinking about it, and after seeing the long term results from all over the world, I believe it has only done good. Because of the title the real message has reached people who would perhaps otherwise never have been touched by it. The way I look at it is this. If this book gets to those people who are 'serial dieters', then that's just great. I know from personal experience that jumping from one diet to another is not a bundle of fun, and if I can do anything to break anyone's diet merry-go-round then I will – no matter what method is required (well, within reason!). My aim is for this to be the last book with the word 'diet' on the cover that they will ever feel the need to buy. And throughout the book you will discover that I never once refer to the 7 lbs in 7 Days programme as a 'diet'; I always use the words 'plan' or 'programme'.

If you are a serial dieter yourself and you feel you have been mislead into thinking this is a seven-day 'diet' and that you will do it and then are able to go back to your old way of eating and drinking, then I make no apologies. I'm up for the challenge. All you need to do is open your mind, read the book and do the programme. I can guarantee you won't be able to give up your new juicy lifestyle after the seven days. Yes, you'll eat again – you cannot live on juice alone, and who on Earth would want to? – but you will not have the same mental urges to go back to your old lifestyle. You will be juiced on both a physical *and* mental level.

Although the programme is entitled 7 lbs in 7 Days, it is not designed solely for people who are overweight. In fact, the programme is one of the best body cleansing programmes on the market today – the ultimate 7-Day Super Detox, if you will. Even if you have no weight to lose I would strongly suggest for the sake of your health and energy levels that you jump on the programme as soon as possible. The only time I would say not to do it is if you are *too* thin. Underweight is a much harder condition to treat than overweight. You would never think, 'I'd rather have a skinny problem than a fat problem,' if you only knew the reality.

*I Cannot Make You **Thin** – but I Can Make You **Slim***

This programme is based on nature's principles, and if you are already a decent weight, don't panic, you won't get 'skinny' doing this. I know some people want to get skinny, but this programme hasn't been designed to turn anyone anorexic! You can make yourself 'thin' by eating three bars of chocolate a day, smoking twenty cigarettes and drinking four vodka and diet cokes a day. Yes, it's true. If that's all you consumed you *would* lose weight and become 'thin', but as you can imagine, a chocolate, fags, booze and diet coke diet would not be a healthy one. Just remember, most heroin addicts are also 'thin'!

What I'm talking about here is finding a good *healthy* system that will enable you either to kick-start a healthy eating lifestyle, give yourself a quick super detox, help with a particular illness, or, for those of you who are overweight (which is the majority), to lose 7 lbs in 7 days in a healthy way.

Since this book was first published I have been searching for ways to make the programme even easier to follow. This is why there is now an app – a full delivery system of the programme direct to your mobile (yes, how cool is that! – see my website for details). It's also why, in this fully updated edition, I have decided to include my handy colour-coded wall planner for the 7-day programme. This has been available to buy separately for a few years and has been an invaluable tool for thousands of people. It contains all the recipes, and is fully colour-coded by the time and method they require. It's a very helpful tool and means that once you have read the book, you no longer need to refer to it to see what you need to do. But please do not make the mistake of just taking out the wall planner, downloading the shopping list from the site and cracking on with the plan. If you do there is a good chance that you will fail – you have been warned! I'm being neither defeatist nor negative, simply realistic – based on my many years of experience. It's essential that you *read the book first!* I'll soon repeat this point in 'The Rules' – and for good reason. If you are not armed with the right frame of mind and a complete understanding of *why* you are juicing rather than just *how* to do it, you will most likely fail. You have been warned – and soon you'll be warned again!

Luckily, the vast majority of people *do* read the book and *do* succeed. This is partly because it's extremely easy to read. Most people read the whole book within a day, some people taking just a couple of hours. Time is precious these days and many people don't have a vast amount of it to spend reading, especially if they want results ... *fast!* Many of the tens of thousands of people who have succeeded on this plan have gone far beyond even what I expected when I first wrote the book.

The letters, calls, e-mails and even video diaries still continue to flood into juicy HQ. When I first wrote the book, I knew from my own experience and others I have helped over the years that the results would be good, but even I wasn't quite prepared for just *how* good. Nor was I quite ready for the often moving, uplifting and life changing messages from people who not only have read the whole book and completed the programme to the letter, but also who *fully* understood the message: fully understood why the programme was designed and how it is a catalyst to a *permanent* slim, trim, healthy body and mind and not just a one-off-drop-a-few pounds 'diet'.

I sincerely hope this book achieves for you what it has for so many people around the world. I also hope that the following small selection of testimonials that I've picked out inspires you to make a point of reading the book and following the programme instead of simply talking about 'doing it one day'. After all:

'*The Road of* **"One Day"** *Leads to a Town Called* **"Never"**'

May the Juice Be with You
Jason Vale

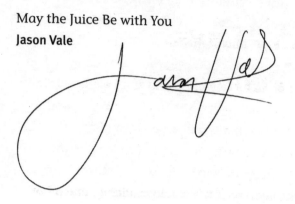

7 lbs in 7 Days:
What People Say

You can have all the scientific data on juicing, and all of the info about what vitamins and minerals are in them, but what really juices people is hard proof. If you are anything like me, you'd like to hear that you are not about to waste your time and energy on something that doesn't get results. You don't want to 'hope' it will make a difference, you want to be certain. The bottom line is

Does It **Work?**

The answer, as you will read from this small sample of testimonials, shows a resounding

YES – It **Does!**

It's worth pointing out to any sceptics that the following testimonials are 100% genuine and unsolicited. The letters and e-mails, which the following are taken from, are available for all to see. I have received thousands of testimonials over the short years this book has been out, here are just a very small sample of what people are saying and the results they are getting.

I sincerely hope you read this little book, follow the programme and reap the truly incredible rewards.

> '*I have just completed your 7lbs in 7 Days plan and want to say how amazed I am at the results – I lost 15lbs! I'm still in absolute shock. I wasn't severely overweight – I was 11 stone 3lbs and am now 10 stone 2lbs. This has now completely inspired me and I have followed on with Turbo-Charge Your Life in 14 Days. Since the birth of my second child I have been eating the wrong foods – chocolate, bread, sweets ... to combat severe exhaustion! And I have found it impossible to shift the weight, but not anymore! Last night was a joy when I managed to get back into my "skinny" jeans! C.'*

> '*Hi, I would just like to say "thank you" ... I found it easy doing juicing for 7 days and I lost 8.2lbs! I started on 29 April and now at my weigh-in this morning, 21 June (nearly 8 weeks later), I weigh 149.2lbs, i.e. 26.8lbs lighter from when I first started with juicing and your plan! I have also lost 5.5% of my body fat and my BMI is down by 4.5. I am writing this to you*

because I thought it may be used to encourage other 70+-year-olds to do something about their diet. Thanks again, J.'

'Hi Jason, before I started the 7lbs in 7 Days Programme I weighed 8st 12lbs. Now I weigh 8 stone and I have stayed at that weight for the last five months. It's great to know that I never have to diet again. I enjoyed the delicious juices so much while doing the programme, I now replace either my breakfast or lunch with a juice. I also start my day around 6.30am on my mini trampoline and I have increased my walking. What I find now is I don't eat biscuits or cakes anymore. I have no desire to put something negative into my body. I don't feel hungry between meals anymore. I have so much energy and I feel so alive and positive. I feel so light, not full of rubbish anymore. Before I started juicing I used to feel so tired and it was an effort to do most things. But those days are gone. Sorry if I have gone on a bit. Anyway thanks again for every thing ... take care and thank you a thousand times!'

'Hi, I am 57 and have had 6 children (including twins). I am a Ballet teacher, and after my first 4 children I was 9½ stone. Since having the twins 25 years ago I have not been under 12 stone. I have tried every diet going but never managed to get under the 12 stone mark. THEN ... A few weeks ago my daughter introduced me to your

*juicing plan. Well .... I have completed the 7 days ...
and lost an AMAZING 11lbs! I couldn't believe it when I
weighed myself, moved the scales and weighed myself
again THREE TIMES, then went next door and borrowed
my neighbour's scales ... and then realised ... IT WAS
TRUE! I am now on day 3 of the Turbo charge in 14 days
and following the book ... I started this plan at 12 stone
10lbs and really want to stick with it until I get to my
proper weight, but I would like to get to under 11 stone
before I go on holiday to Italy in 2 weeks. I am now 11
stone 13lbs! ... Many thanks.'*

*'I am absolutely over the moon, I just can't believe it. I
knew I'd lost weight but I'd never dreamt it possible
that I could lose an overwhelming 9.6 lbs in just 7 days,
it's amazing! Thank you so very much.'*

*'I'm amazed, I have not only lost 8.2 lbs on the 7-day
Super Juice programme, I have also lost 2 inches from
my waist and hips! On top of that, I also did the Turbo
plan and lost a further 8½ lbs. The thing that surprised
me most was that I never felt uncomfortably hungry
and to my further amazement I could only manage an
average of three juices a day. I thought I'd easily not
only have all five, but would be wanting much more.
Although I missed my cup of decaf tea on the
programme, I was surprised to see that although I
could have one after the programme, I didn't want to!*

'The best side effect is the way you feel. I never thought that changing your diet could have such a profound effect on your mental state. I guess you really are what you eat – thank you. X'

'To have lost over 9 lbs in just 7 days is so rewarding and is such a huge incentive for anyone looking to try this plan. In this day and age we all want to see instant results, we want it NOW! And with this plan you can get it!'

'This programme has been an absolute win, win, win. I've spent less time and money on shopping, it's just so simple as there's no deliberating on what to buy, or scanning packets for calorie content, or calculating points values, or assessing GI indexes – its just so simple and it works, it really, really works! Thank you.'

'I just feel so fantastic, I feel lighter mentally and physically and I'm full of energy. I didn't think it possible to lose so much weight without being hungry and at the same time know you're giving your body everything it needs in terms of nutrition.'

The Rules

I would like to make something clear before we start. As the testimonials above suggest, what you are about to read has the power not only to reshape your body but also, as a knock-on effect, the ability to reshape many aspects of your life.

Before we start, in order to make this programme work to its maximum potential there are a few ground rules which I need to cover. Please note that these rules are *essential* for the success of the programme.

➤ Read the *entire* book in the order it was written.
➤ Follow the 7-day programme to the letter.
➤ Read at least four pages of the book a day to keep up momentum.
➤ Let Your Mind Be Free.
➤ Follow the Rules!

RULE 1: Read the Entire Book in the Order It Was Written

The first rule is one which I lay down in all of my books. My books are specifically intended to be read in the order they were written – not as a 'flick through' or 'dip in' type of book – and they have been designed to be read in their entirety. It is incredible the number of people who buy books of this nature and either don't read them at all or just 'flick through' the pages. This book will only be effective if you read it in the order it has been written. *Flicking through this book will not give you the results you are looking for.*

I am fully aware that some of you will feel you have a race against time at the moment (perhaps you have a wedding, a party or a date coming up) and you want to skip the reading and just do the programme. However, the 'pre-plan' is extremely important and the wise saying of 'less haste more speed' is never more apt than here. Clearly, you can just jump ahead. After all, you can attempt to cross a road away from a designated crossing zone during rush hour, blindfolded and with your legs tied together. But the chances of your getting to the other side in one piece would be a good deal smaller than if you crossed *without* your legs tied and *without* the blindfold at a pelican crossing. Equally, this programme can be done without any mental preparation, but the chances of true success are next to none. These few rules are here for a reason. You have been warned!

RULE 2: Follow the 7-Day Programme to the Letter!

If you follow Rule 1, Rule 2 will follow naturally. To reiterate, the programme will be MUCH easier if you follow Rule 1 *before* you jump into the programme.

RULE 3: Read at Least 4 Pages of the Book Each Day to Keep up Momentum

Momentum is without question the key. This rule is just as important as the other two. How many times have you started something – a book, a language course, an exercise programme, a change of eating programme – only to find that other things soon got in the way and you never finished it? By following the rule of reading at least four pages a day, come whatever, you will achieve something that over 90% of people who buy books of this nature fail to achieve. You will actually finish the book you have bought. What a concept!

RULE 4: Let Your Mind Be Free

An open or, as I like to say, *free* mind is of paramount importance when reading this book. We tend to carry so much baggage in our heads that we are rarely free to accept new information, new opportunities, new ideas. We tend to have an extremely entrenched view of what is correct on many subjects – none more so than on the subject of health and nutrition – and we tend to believe that what we know is absolute fact.

The chances of this being the only book you have read on the subject of health/diet and nutrition are very slight, not to mention the numerous TV shows you have probably watched. It is likely you will have accumulated a great deal of information that you now regard as fact, and if you read anything in this book which contradicts this information, you may find it easy to dismiss it.

All I ask you is that you allow your mind to be free – especially when it comes to my style of writing. My style isn't for everyone. We are all different and the old saying, 'You can please all of the people some of the time but you cannot please all of the people all of the time,' is particularly appropriate here. Not all of you reading this book will like the way I put things, my attempts at humour, my mild swearing at times, or my constant repetition of key points. However, everything I write is here for a reason. And, trust me; there is no way I would ever want to write more than is absolutely necessary. The repetition of key points is vital in order to get the essential message beyond your conscious into your subconscious. Although this may 'jar' with you at times and you may feel it unnecessary, please allow your mind to be open to this approach.

Fortunately, most people like my no-nonsense, tell-it-like-it-is, chatty approach, and find my books incredibly easy and often funny to read. This is a conscious and deliberate approach on my part as it makes completing Rule 1 – Read the Entire Book in the Order It Was Written – so much easier to achieve. The most common comment I get from people who write to me or approach me in the streets is: 'It's the only book I've ever read from cover to cover since I've left school.'

You will soon see that I'm not here to win any literary awards. It's just that I have a message and a plan that will get you really juiced.

RULE 5: Follow the Rules

This would appear self-evident and could even be seen as somewhat patronizing, but you'd be amazed at just how many people decide to do something their way – despite whatever the rules or instructions suggest!

If someone was to give you precise instructions for you to able to get from where you are to where you want to be on a road journey, you would be unlikely to take a left when the instructions clearly state right. Equally, if you decide to skip any of the rules or instructions on the programme you will, in all likelihood, end up in a completely different place than you want to be on the slim/health/energy front. If that happens then shouts of 'It didn't work' will rear their ugly head.

IT does work; *IT* will give you the results you are looking for ... but only if *you do IT.*

It is very seldom that 'IT' fails us, rather we fail IT. Very rarely does IT not work for us, rather we don't work for IT.

Follow the rules, follow the instructions and you can be 100% sure that IT will work for you.

Those Were the Rules
... On with the Programme

*'Life **shrinks** or*
***expands** in proportion*
to one's courage'

Anaïs Nin

Are You Ready to
E X P A N D
Your World?
Let's begin ...

1

Totally Juiced in Just 7 Days!

The following programme – if you do it to the letter – will give you startling results on the health and weight-loss front in just 168 hours. Not only will you drop an average of 7 lbs in just 7 days, but more importantly than that, you will do so in an extremely healthy way and your energy levels will really go through the roof. Not only will you lose the weight, but also – provided you have followed the Rules – you will be in the right mind set be able to keep the weight off *permanently*. Put simply, the results that people are getting on this unique programme are being described as nothing short of remarkable.

This isn't simply rhetoric, wishful thinking or 'hyping it up'; it is *precisely* what happens to people who complete the 7-Day Super Juice programme.

The testimonials at the start are just a taster of the sort of life-expanding, body-shrinking results people are achieving. Yes, people do get slimmer on this programme, with most people dropping *more* than 7 lbs. However, because they are doing this using the power of the finest and most nutritious liquid fuel on the planet – bar none – and because this book deals with the mental side as well as the physical, they also experience many other incredible changes to how they look and feel. I have seen almost every common aliment improve, or in some cases, completely disappear with the help of this programme. At my 7lbs In 7 Days Super Juice Detox Retreat in Turkey, I have seen people arrive with life-long health problems and leave without them – in just seven days. We should never underestimate the power of the body to heal itself when given the right nutrients and opportunity to do so. The two biggest causes of all disease are 'toxicity' and 'deficiency'. This unique programme removes the toxicity and addresses any nutrient deficiency. However, for most people doing this programme getting amazing health will simply come about as a side-effect of their real desired outcome – a flat stomach!

Let's Be **Politically** Correct ...
Or Maybe **Not!**

When we cut through all the politically correct nonsense as to why most people ever go on a programme of this nature, the hard truth is it comes down to two basic human desires:

1 We want to **look** bloody good.
2 We want to **feel** bloody good.

That's it!

Yes, we can all say, 'I'm doing this because I want to be healthy, I don't want to die young and I want to be a good role model for my kids' – all of which may very well be true. But the bottom line is that the vast majority of us jump on a programme like this because we want to look sexy, feel vibrant and alive and, if we are being brutally honest, YES, God damn it, we also want that flat stomach! Not only do we want it, almost crave it, but, as is the way of our super-fast 21st-century world, we want to look and feel amazing in the fastest possible time – in other words, RIGHT NOW! I know this is not the done thing to say and yes we all should aim for 'steady weight loss', but if we cut through all the bull, we all want amazing results on the slim and trim front and we want those results NOW!

Quick-Fix Dangers ... but Not on This Programme

The danger with the 'I want to see my stomach muscles before tomorrow morning'-type approach to weight loss and looking good is that it usually involves a drastic *unhealthy* system that will, in the long run, cause the body's metabolism to slow down so much that it will inevitably cause you to gain *more* weight when you eventually start eating normally again.

In 1983, diet 'guru' Geoffrey Cannon wrote a book titled *Dieting Makes You Fat*. This is based on the theory that when your body is starved of all food and nutrients it goes into famine mode. And when the body is in famine mode, guess what it needs to hang on to most of all for its source of energy? Yep – FAT! Not only that but he also stated that the more that people go on a strict 'where's my food gone' type of diet, the *more* their bodies will protect the stores of fat, thus making it more difficult to lose weight the next time. In 1986, a study carried out on a group of rats showed that by the time they had gone through their second diet, the weight loss was half what it had been the first time – and the weight was put back on three times as fast!

This is why I'm very excited to bring you this programme. Not only has it been carefully designed to nourish your body completely on a cellular level – meaning you will *not* be starving yourself – but I have also added the right psychology for success *and* a plan for the following weeks. This is to make sure you introduce the right foods gradually, so as not to shock your system, *and* I have also included a 'guideline for life' plan which will allow your body to continue to lose weight (*if required*) and, more importantly, not put it back on.

No *Brainer*

This is where most 'lose a few pounds' programmes fall flat on their faces. They usually consist of a 7-, 14- or 21-day super plan which is based on an unsound nutritional programme, no mental preparation whatsoever and nowhere to go afterwards. It tends to be a case of 'You've done your seven days [or whatever], now go back to eating the same crap as you were before,' which makes very little sense. It is this approach that creates the whole diet merry-go-round.

The problem is not so much that people start to eat normally again after a detox/slim/health programme, but more the problem lies in what their idea of 'normal' is!

This is what bugs me about some dieticians and doctors. They group all 'diets' together as one and say, 'Once a person starts eating normally again after a "crash diet" they will regain the weight they've lost – and much more on top.' But surely the problem arises with the use of the word 'normally'. Wasn't it their 'normal' diet which made people who go on diets fat to start with? Surely that means unless these people change their idea of what 'normal' is they will always gain weight again. Not because of the 'diet' but because they go back to *their* 'normal' amount of food.

I have received thousands of e-mails from people from all over the world who have not only lost the initial 7lbs but, because the book and the programme in it helped to change their mindset, have gone on to lose *all* of their excess weight because the programme became a lifestyle for them. In other words, they managed to change what their idea of 'normal' was. Because they read the book, understood the message and did the entire plan, they now eat 'normally' all the time. When you do that, you keep the weight off. It's only when you eat *abnormally* that you will become obese.

It will come as no surprise that I'm not into the 'Get Slim Quick' approach, and anyone who has read my first book *Slim For Life: Freedom from the Food Trap* or the bestselling *The Juice Master: Turbo-Charge Your Life in 14 Days* will know this already. I'm into lifestyle change, *mind* change, a change that lasts – no quick fixes to the detriment of future weight and health.

However, I'm also aware that people want to see results ... *FAST!* And I'm also aware that sometimes quick results can create unbelievable momentum for people – momentum that can lead to amazing future success on the health and fitness front.

The Price Is Right

In 2005 I was asked if I would put together a nutrition plan for Katie Price (yes, the famous model Jordan). Katie had never been near a juice extractor in her life and was living on a diet consisting of nothing but take-aways and fast food such as pizza and McDonald's. Katie had been pretty lucky on the weight front most of her life. Despite her awful diet and no exercise, her system managed to keep her slim – even springing back to its flat stomach self *immediately* after the birth of her first child, Harvey.

However, despite what people may think, Katie wasn't so
fortunate after her second child. She needed a caesarean
and even after the baby was born she still had 28lbs to
lose! Contrary to popular rumour, Katie did not have a
tummy tuck, and from what I now know of her she never
would. Isn't it amazing what people make up to make
themselves feel better!

Like most women who have recently given birth she had
weight to lose, and like most she wanted to lose it in super-
fast time. Her main reason for wanting to lose the weight
fast – as well as her work as a model – was her impending
wedding. Katie, like most brides to be, wanted to look
amazing for the day, and even though she had three
months to lose the weight she wanted some results *fast*.

I devised a specific six-week juicing/eating plan and
explained that as it was new to her it would take a short
time to get used to juicing; it would also take time to lose
the weight but to be patient and her body would do what it
needed to do.

Asking Katie to be patient is like asking Jim Carrey to
keep still! She is a woman who wants results in the fastest
possible time and the initial plan wasn't producing
changes quick enough for her. At this stage people often do
one of two things. They either go back to what they were
eating before – which clearly doesn't help their cause – or
they do something incredibly drastic like living on nothing
but water and doing four hours' exercise a day; again far
from good and far from being in the same ball park as
healthy.

This is when I suggested she went on *nothing* but specially designed juices and smoothies for 7 days. I explained that the average person loses 7lbs on the programme, that it is extremely healthy, but it requires a great deal of preparation and a certain mind set in order to achieve it. But I didn't realize at the time who I was dealing with. Katie is perhaps the most determined person I have ever met and if she says she's going to do something she will do it whatever it takes to make sure it gets done.

I would say Katie kept to the programme 90–95% of the time and saw some great results at the end of that week. More importantly, she now knew that there was indeed something to this juicing lark as she wasn't anywhere near as hungry as she thought she would be and often not hungry at all. This, along with the dramatic weight loss, gave her the momentum to continue to Phases 2 and 3 of the programme. (These phases are included in this programme to make sure the change sticks.)

Katie not only lost the weight she wanted to lose but, much more than that, *she has kept it off*. At the time of writing this book, some three months after she finished her juice plan with me, Katie is weighing in at an average of 8 stone (106lbs). This would be way too thin for some, but for Katie's height and frame it's a perfectly healthy weight. And as I write this fully updated version of the book some five years later, Katie still weighs an average of 106lbs.

The point I want to make is that having juice as part of her daily diet is not a diet to her; it is now a lifestyle, and without it the chances are she would still be on a diet consisting largely of take-aways. As she says:

> 'This is the first time I have ever stuck to any sort of diet plan ... I love the juices and I don't feel hungry.'

This is why I make no apologies for this perfectly healthy, amazing results, super juice plan. If it juices people to initiate life-long changes and embark on a healthier lifestyle, then I'm all for it.

I have told Katie's story as her body, health and weight are often in the media. But nearly all of the most amazing juicy stories are from 'regular' people.

Not Such a Regular Guy

I remember a guy coming on one of my 'Health Weekends' who arrived *very* sceptical, left *very* sceptical and – if it weren't for the rapid results he achieved after doing a specially devised '8-day challenge' when he left the weekend – probably would have remained sceptical ... *and fat!* This man was about 250lbs when I met him; he is now just over 170lbs! That's a massive, massive, change. It's the difference of being able to walk without a constant chafing on your inner thighs; it's the difference of being able to run and play; it's the difference of being able to go into a shop and buy whatever clothes you like; it's the difference of being able to get into a bathing costume without the constant paranoia that everyone and their mother is looking at and judging you. This man is happier than ever, more passionate about life than he has been in years, has much more energy – and he looks good! This is the power of what juice can do and the power of seeing good results in a short space of time; it can boost you into major life change *and* inspire you to continue. This is why it worked for Jordan, the guy you just read about and thousands of others for whom good fast results on the juice programme have enabled them to have faith in juicing, continue to do it and now have a very juicy lifestyle. And it is why it can work for you.

It's all well and good telling people to 'be patient' when they change what they eat and that the 'body will drop the weight when it is ready', but that is hardly going to help you fit into that little black dress or tuck into those jeans in time to party!

Yes, I'm being slightly facetious, but no matter how much we try to cover it up or ignore it, the fact is that this is no longer a world where patience prevails. Whether we like it or not, the instant gratification society has taken over in what can only be described as a ...

2

Super-fast World

We live in a world of fast cars, fast trains, fast planes, fast TV, fast games; we eat super fast, drink fast, speak fast and of course – the big one – we have plenty of fast food. We also live in a world where change in technology happens in a nanosecond. Where we were once amazed that it is possible to communicate and send pictures over the Internet, nowadays if our computer doesn't do what we want in two seconds flat, we'll start swearing at the blooming thing in no time.

We live in a world where we want, *and expect*, super-fast results with everything – including weight loss and improved health. This is why if there is a safe, highly nutritious way that will enable people to see quick results, then I'm all for it. Especially when the likelihood is they will then get so juiced and excited by what they see that they'll continue with Phases 2 and Phase 3 of the programme.

Clearly not everyone will continue with the Juicy Lifestyle; I'm a realist, and many will simply use the 7-day programme as a quick, 'Oh, Bugger me, I have to look good for the wedding/party/date/holiday/boy/girl/ whatever – and I have to do it fast!' But that's OK. The worst thing that will happen is that you will give your body a super cleanse, lose some weight, feel good and get healthier – and what's wrong with that? What's wrong with someone who usually eats a diet full of crap drinking some powerful liquid fuel for a week and giving their body a much-needed rest?

Equally, many people will use this system specifically as a 'super health clean' – almost like putting their body in for service once every three months. In fact, going on this programme once every season is one of the best things you can ever do for your health and even your longevity – and again this isn't hearsay.

Twice the Life

Dr Roy Walford has written five books on the subject of immunology and ageing. Based on his numerous long-term experiments, he is convinced that the human lifespan should be 120 years and we should arrive there virtually free of disease. There are a few cultures around the world, such as the Hunzacut tribe, who do in fact live that long, thus perhaps semi-proving Dr Walford's point. However, what interested me in particular was his work on mice. The normal lifespan of mice is about two years, yet Dr

Walford's mice live an average of twice that long. How does he achieve this amazing feat? All he does is give the mice their normal food for five days of the week and then just water for the remaining two days. In other words, he simply rests their digestive systems for 48 hours every week and the mice live TWICE as long.

Now clearly I am not suggesting you will live twice as long if you did this, but I am suggesting that you can have twice the life while you *are* here.

When you stop burdening your body with energy-zapping, life-depleting 'foods' and drinks, it not only has a huge impact on the actual length of time you will live, but more importantly, when your system is clean, your mind is clearer and your spirits are higher; all of this will lead to you wanting to experience more of what life has to offer and so in turn having more of a life. And I'm not suggesting that by doing this programme once or even four times a year that you will slow down the ageing process either. In fact, while I'm about it I want to get this off my chest:

You Cannot **Slow** Down the **Ageing** Process

Yes, there are creams and lotions that claim they can slow down the process and, yes, on the surface you can appear younger, but that doesn't mean you actually are! Appearances can be deceiving, and just because you are looking good on the outside because of a few face-tightening creams, the surgeon's knife or bathing in asses' milk, it doesn't mean for one second that your internal organs are as young as your external self.

Equally, there are no foods on the planet that can help slow down the ageing process. All you naturopaths out there reading this may well be shouting at the book in the strong belief that there are indeed many foods provided by nature that will slow down the ageing process. However, it's only us humans and the animals that *we* feed who seem to die at such differing ages. We are also the only creatures on the planet whose regular diet essentially consists of denatured food and we are also the only ones on the planet who overburden their digestive system on a regular basis and who consume God knows how much alcohol a week.

Caffeine, nicotine, refined sugars and fats, stress, drugs and a defeatist frame of mind have all been linked to *speeding* up the ageing process. But when you stop doing one, a few or all of these things you don't slow down the ageing process – you just stop speeding it up. There is a big difference between the two.

So it's not that the raw power of freshly extracted fruits and vegetables plus a few Super Food supplements in this programme will help to slow down the ageing process, it's just that the rate at which you age will be slower than it would have been had you been eating and drinking rubbish.

We Are Not Living *Longer* We Are Surviving *Longer*

Many doctors and dieticians argue that historically we are now living longer than ever, but the reality is we are surviving longer, not living longer. There is a massive difference between just getting through the day and then collapsing in a heap in front of the TV, and truly living. There are many people in their 50s, 60s, 70s and 80s who may well be alive in the sense that their heart is still ticking, but who actually stopped truly living long ago. Hang on! What am I talking about here? I know many people in their 20s, 30s and 40s who stopped living years ago, let alone people in their 60s or 70s. I know people in their 20s, 30s and 40s who aren't just feeling fat, lethargic and depressed, but who actually feel old!

> '*If you think you are old you are right,* *if you **don't** think you are old* *you are **also** right*'

'*How Old Would You Be, If You Didn't Know How Old You Are?*'
Leroy (Satchel) Paige

Life breeds life, and if you are constantly stressing your digestive system with too many of the wrong sorts of foods and drinks there is no question you will feel, and therefore *be*, older than you are. There is also no question that the physical side effects of a bad diet and no exercise, such as being overweight and lacking in energy, can often shatter your courage and lower your spirits. And low spirits age someone quicker than anything else.

This is why I have specifically devised this plan with fast, *healthy* results in mind. As I mentioned, like it or not, we all want instant gratification, and I know that cleaning out the system with nature's super juices and seeing startling results in super-fast time can lift someone's spirits like almost nothing else and thus give them a zest for life again. Yes, a sign of affection from the people we love should be enough to make our day, and clearly it can help a great deal, but if we are being honest, for many people there's nothing quite like the feeling of fitting into those jeans to lift the spirits!

This is why I love the fact that with this programme there is such a difference on the weight and energy levels in super-fast time. The letters, e-mails and video diaries I have received from those who have done the programme have shown not only a great difference in body aesthetics, but more importantly in spirit. It is spirit that keeps us alive; it is spirit that drives us; it is spirit that makes us want to get out of bed and live as opposed to survive; and it is spirit that makes us want to better ourselves, our lives and enrich the people around us.

This is why very, very few people simply do the 7-day programme and then go back to their old lifestyles. Most people who do the programme are so juiced by the end of the 7 days that they continue and do the Phase 2 Turbo-Charge and Phase 3 Juicy Lifestyle plans. The average weight loss on the 7-day Juice Plan is about 8 lbs, but combined with the 2-week Turbo Plan the average weight loss in the 21 days is an amazing 18 lbs!

However, despite the fact we are in an obese epidemic and despite all of what I've said, I can still hear some people shouting ...

3

'But It's Never Healthy to Lose Weight Fast'

Well, when I said I can still hear people saying, 'But it's never healthy to lose weight fast,' I meant many doctors and dieticians. When talking to dieticians, nutritionists and doctors about this 7-day Super Juice programme, I was continually hit by the same old rhetoric:

> *'Yes, the person may lose 7 lbs in 7 days, but some of that will be water and maybe even tissue, it won't all be fat.'*

This may well be true, to some extent – *although not in every case* – but if it gets us into that little black dress, or gets our six-pack showing, what the hell do we care! OK, so now I am being factious. Yes, we do care and, yes, we do want to lose fat and, yes, we don't want our muscles to waste away and, yes, we want to be healthy, but hey, as I've mentioned, we also want to look good ... *fast!* They then go on:

*'... and a weight loss fast of this nature can never be
healthy and will inevitably result in the person
becoming fatter in the long run.'*

Really?

Well, firstly it's not a fast. I hate it when I hear of people describing this plan as a 'juice fast'. It's a contradiction in terms. You cannot be fasting while you are having freshly extracted juices. A fast is where a person drinks only water and takes in no nutrients from food whatsoever. Juicing furnishes the body with the finest, easiest to ingest nutrients on the planet, and juicing retains 95% of the nutrients in fruit and vegetables. Let me reiterate that:

Juicing Retains **95%** of the Nutrients in **Fruits** and **Vegetables**

And given these highly charged macro- and micro-nutrients are often much more bio-available to your cells (meaning more of the nutrients will get to where they are needed), there is no way on Earth that this programme can be described as a fast.

Secondly, it's ironic that any programme that feeds every cell in the body with precisely what it requires for optimum health could possibly be called unhealthy. I laugh out loud when people tell me that this programme is not only unhealthy but, wait for it – dangerous. Yes, DANGEROUS! I kid you not. This programme has actually been described by a few uninformed doctors and dieticians

– the very people who are meant to be in charge of our nation's health and vitality – as dangerous. Now call me Mr Are You Flipping Kidding Me, but how on Earth can ridding yourself of junk food, caffeine, alcohol and other crap from your diet and pouring in nature's finest super foods for a week be described in any way, shape or form as dangerous?

This gets my goat more than anything else. I feel like shouting out, 'LOOK, THESE PEOPLE WERE FAT AND ILL AND NEEDED HELP!' I feel like yelling, 'LOOK AT THESE PEOPLE, THEY'RE JUST ONE MORE CREAM BUN AWAY FROM DIABETES, HEART DISEASE, A STROKE, EVEN CANCER!'

Diabetes was relatively unheard of when I was growing up. Now we are in a situation where 1.8 million people in the UK have diabetes – that's a 450% increase from 1960. And this is just the people who know about it. It is estimated that at least 1 million more have diabetes but don't know it. The UK has the fastest-growing rate of diabetes in Europe, along with the fastest-growing rate of obesity. Globally, cases of diabetes have risen from 55 million in 1955 to 150 million in 2004, and are projected to grow to 300 million by 2025. In the UK alone the projected figure is 3 million confirmed sufferers within the next six years. This isn't some slightly inconvenient disease either: type 2 diabetes (the most common) causes more amputations a year than even smoking-related diseases. Yes, amputations! On top of that, diabetes is directly responsible for many losing their sight. Diabetes can make you blind!

Heart disease has now overtaken cancer as the nation's biggest killer and, like diabetes, very few cases are hereditary and **nearly all cases are caused directly by what we eat and drink!** Even the World Health Organization admits:

85% of Western Disease is Caused Directly by What We Put into Our Mouth

Given these facts, I just cannot understand why any doctor or dietician would be against anyone going from a diet of rubbish to one of nature's pure super foods or why they might even consider it to be dangerous. You would think all doctors would love an approach to weight loss which only involved nature's finest healing foods and didn't involve a drug of some description. One reviewer, a well-known dietician who writes for a national newspaper, went so far as to claim that the diet is not only nutritionally questionable but also makes anyone who practises it hungry and unhappy.

However, my research – which involves thousands of real people who have given their feedback on my juice programme – suggests otherwise.

Here are a couple of examples:

> *'I started at 14 stone 3lbs and weighed in a fantastic 13 stone 7lbs – an amazing 10lbs loss in just 7 days. Brilliant, amazing, incredible! All those words and more. I cannot thank Jason enough for developing*

*such an amazing plan. I have gone on to your next
stages and have lost almost 2 stone in 8 weeks. People
are absolutely gobsmacked when I tell them and they
can't get enough information about how it all works.
Two of my colleagues have already bought the book
and lost 7lbs and 10lbs respectively. Sincere thanks, a
verrrrry happy C.'*

C was 199lbs in weight and within eight weeks of reading
the book he was 28lbs lighter. How on earth is that either
dangerous or the sign of a man who is feeling miserable
and can't wait to eat crap again, given that he signed off
'thanks, a verrrrry happy C'?

Here's another piece of correspondence that I hope
doctors and dieticians read. It illustrates the power of rapid
weight loss on one's mind:

*'This programme is a lifesaver ... there's simply no
other way to describe it. I'm hooked and believe me, if I
can do it, anyone can do it. The truth is when you get
quick results, your motivation is sky-rocketed and you
can see a light at the end of what was once a very dark
tunnel. I've lost as much weight in the first four days as
I did in four weeks on my last "diet", where I felt
deprived, discouraged and frankly defeated. Thank
you, thank you, thank you! D.'*

These are just two of thousands of examples of people who
have either shed loads of weight and kept it off, or who

have seen impressive results quickly that have inspired them to continue. I have known people to lose over 100lbs in weight after reading my book. Lord Harris of Peckham, no less, lost 42lbs in just three weeks and dropped three points from his cholesterol after reading the book. Quick, *healthy* weight loss, *along with the right frame of mind*, inspires people to long-term good health and weight loss – IT IS NOT DANGEROUS!

What *is* dangerous is *not* taking action, *not* changing your lifestyle, *not* changing your diet. What *is* dangerous, I feel, are the countless dieticians and doctors who constantly tell people it's not healthy to lose more than 2lbs a week because it's been scientifically backed up. It was also scientifically backed up that smoking helped to relax you! Science isn't always what it's cracked up to be. If you weigh 200lbs and you lose 2lbs in a week, you don't feel good. You don't feel inspired to continue. You don't feel fired up. More often than not, you will fail at your diet. It's madness that when I'm on the Shopping Channel they're not even allowed to show the front cover of this book. Why not? Because dieticians and their kind have somehow convinced the watchdogs that losing 7lbs in 7 days is dangerous. They have managed to do this while we have the most serious obesity crisis in history. The world has officially gone bonkers.

What is also very dangerous, in my opinion, are the people in charge of advising us on health describing a programme such as this as dangerous whilst handing out anti-obesity drugs at the same time. These drugs, let's not forget, often hit the front pages of newspapers due to the often horrific side effects. The day I read a front-page headline reporting new research that shows fruit and vegetables to be bad for us is the day I pack all this in and start agreeing with the 'if they're ill give 'em a pill' culture. Until that day, I'll follow Hippocrates' advice:

> '*Of several remedies, the physician should choose the least sensational.*'

This then is perhaps the biggest irony. Some doctors say that it is dangerous to have a 'quick fix' attitude to weight loss and health, while this is precisely what they try to achieve with the drugs they hand out so liberally. After all, instant gratification is precisely what the medical drug culture is built on. For years most of the medical profession has handed out antibiotics like Smarties for ailments such as flu – a virus against which antibiotics do *nothing*. Let's not forget that since 'obesity' has been classed as a disease in its own right, the fight by drug companies to get their all-singing, all-dancing, anti-fat pills on the market has been fierce.

Big people are Big Business to the pharmaceutical industry, and it seems they will do anything to sell their wares to their customers. And their customers are not so much the obese patients themselves, but the thousands of doctors whom they have to convince to prescribe their new wonder drug. Even if some dreadful side effect rears its ugly head during the development stages, it appears it is often explained away as 'incidental to the greater good of the drug'. It is only when people start getting problems like anal leakage – as was the case with the anti-fat drug Xenical – that questions are asked. It appears that anti-fat drugs which have been known to have even worse side effects than Xenical are OK when it's the greater good that's in question, but a programme such as the one in this book gets hammered by the medical industry. And this is a programme that relies purely on nature's healing principles; one which does nothing to tax the liver and one that has no adverse side effects.

I'm certainly not saying that medical drug intervention isn't absolutely necessary at times, or that it never does any good, as clearly it does and many lives are saved as a result. I know this first hand as I was badly asthmatic and needed my blue Ventolin inhaler up to sixteen times a day – trust me, that little blue inhaler was my lifesaver. However, why do they appear never to suggest we should, as Hippocrates famously did, 'Let food be thy medicine and let thy medicine be food'? Why isn't diet always the *first* thing to be suggested when it comes to any illness? When I changed my diet and started juicing, the first thing to change was my asthma. I went from being unable to survive without my Ventolin inhaler to not needing it at all. I haven't had asthma since. Was this a coincidence? I don't think so!

I also lost weight, my energy levels increased, my nails got stronger, my eyes brighter and my severe psoriasis, which covered my body from head to foot, started to improve *massively*. These incredible health changes occurred with no pills, potions, drugs or medical lotions. They occurred naturally, a concept which, while often lost on some parts of the medical and dietetic profession, is easily explained by means of …

4

The Goldfish Bowl

'The germ is nothing, the terrain is everything.'
Louis Pasteur

Imagine a goldfish in a bowl of clean water. What would happen to the fish if the water was never cleaned? What would happen if the fish was left to live in a polluted environment day after day with the pollution getting slightly worse each day? I think you'd agree that it's likely the fish would probably get an ailment or two.

The question I have is a simple one: What would you do to help the fish? Would you treat the fish or clean the water? Would you give the fish a drug to help with its condition or would you clean the water? You really don't need six years of medical training to come up with the only logical answer:

CLEAN THE FLIPPING WATER!

I'm not saying you should never treat the fish as well; after all, the likelihood is that after years of swimming around in all that pollution it is bound to be unwell. So by all means help the fish by treating it with a pill or whatever – but only as long as you CLEAN THE WATER AT THE SAME TIME! I cannot say this enough; when it comes to health the answer cannot be put more simply:

CLEAN THE WATER!

It amazes me when a doctor sees someone who is obese and then does a load of tests to check on their health. Being overweight is now classed as a disease in its own right – it's when the body is at dis-*ease* with itself. If you saw a group of squirrels and in amongst the group there was a really fat one, I don't somehow think you need to be Dr Sherlock to work out that something was very wrong. You would also know the cause of the problem would have been **too many nuts** – not rocket science. Equally, when you see someone who is massively obese you don't need to take a load of tests to see that they're ill or what the probable cause is.

This is why I find it very hard to keep a straight face when watching Dr Gillian McKeith. All of her TV clients seem to be men and women who eat nothing but junk food and who are as big as a house. She asks them to provide her with a sample stool (poo) which she then analyses to see if they are unwell. I don't mean to be funny but I really don't think you need to look at and smell their crap in order to diagnose that they are facing an enormous number of health problems. You don't need to take a bunch of medical tests or to look at their shit to see quite clearly that they are ill and exactly what the cause is. You also don't need a PhD in medical science to figure out what to do in order to make them better: CLEAN THE WATER. In fact, if you think about it that's all Gillian does. Her clients have polluted systems, so she advises them to cut out the pollution and eat high-water-content, nutrient-packed food. She even actively encourages juicing, as she, like so many more these days, now realizes it is by far the quickest and most nutritious way to clean out the rubbish.

Medical versus Alternative?

If you had a scale and at one end you had the medical profession and at the other end you had the 'alternative therapies', then I guess I'm positioned pretty much in the middle. This isn't me sitting on the fence, it's just I that I can see there are times when both are perfectly justifiable.

Many people in the conventional medical profession instantly rubbish any 'alternative' methods, and equally many people in complementary medicine do the same for drug therapy. In fact, many alternative practitioners have the belief that you should NEVER treat yourself with any medical drugs and that conventional medical treatment is *never* necessary and that all drugs are toxic and cause disease. But somehow I don't think any 'alternative' practitioner, if they had their leg severed in an accident, would think that dissolving a homeopathic tablet under their tongue or inserting an acupuncture needle is going to do the job.

Of course, while medical intervention is necessary *at times,* common sense should tell everyone that for the most part it is *very short-term* medical intervention that is necessary. What is nonsensical is *only* feeding the fish and *never* cleaning the water, which is what happens 99% of the time with conventional medicine and its approach to disease. What is also nonsensical is using any type of approach other than nature's healing liquid foods to treat pretty much all disease, *especially* in someone who is overweight and lethargic.

Half Ton Man

The heaviest recorded man on the planet weighed the same as seven baby elephants! There was even a TV programme made about him entitled *Half Ton Man.* He had been in bed for seven years (that's a pretty big lie-in!). He eventually had medical intervention and lost half his body weight by the time the programme had been broadcast. On the surface it appears that medical intervention was the *only* way forward, but was it? Firstly, who the hell was bringing him the food? I mean, it wasn't as if he could nip out to a fast food joint. Instead of the medical profession taking down half of his house, using a whale hoist to remove him from his bed and take him to hospital, it would have been better to make an order that no junk food whatsoever be brought to him and make it a *criminal* offence if they did. OK, this may seem over the top, but by bringing this man whatever he wanted on the food front, it could be argued that the doctors were assisting a suicide. Why didn't they just feed him freshly extracted juices and smoothies? Why was the 'Clean the Water' type of approach never *forcefully* prescribed?

Being overweight is often simply a symptom of pollution and toxins within the body. When we cut out the rubbish and feed our cells nature's finest in an extremely easy-to-digest form, what we are effectively doing is cleaning the environment in which our cells bathe. As the 'live' nutrients are in a liquid form they are delivered to exactly where they are needed, in super-fast time. This highly charged liquid not only channels the super rich nutrients to the cells, but it also helps flush the system of excess pollution, toxins and FAT! As digestion requires more nerve energy than almost anything else (which is why you fall asleep after a big meal), the juice extractor and blender effectively do the hard work so your system doesn't have to. This energy is saved for the task of removing fat and generally cleaning up and repairing the entire system, making juicing the most effective and healthy way of 'cleaning the water', while at the same time giving life to the system.

> *'The physician should not treat the disease but the patient who is suffering from it.'*
> **Maimonides**

This is also why the results from the 7-day plan go way beyond simply losing 7 lbs. One of the main reasons people are reporting improvements with aliments from IBS to CFS is because we're not talking about some powdered drink you add milk to which is full of artificial sweeteners and other chemicals. What we have is nature's finest ingredients all blended together in their natural 'live' state. No added sugar, salt, fat, chemicals, E numbers, stabilizers or anything artificial, just pure natural liquid fuel injecting life into every one of your cells – liquid fuel that is loaded with amino acids, natural carbohydrates, beneficial fats, vitamins, minerals, water and enzymes.

The simple truth is that once you stop the pollution, put life back into the system and 'clean the water', all of a sudden weight loss and health miracles start to happen effortlessly. I know it sounds too simple, but then why need it be complicated?

Intuitive Doctoring

Nature already provides us with the most effective self-doctoring mechanism known to wo/mankind – *instinct*. Instinctively, everyone who reads this book knows that it makes perfect sense. Instinctively, it is impossible to argue against nature and her incredible ability to heal with foods specifically designed for us. The problem is that we have been brought up in such a 'you must treat the fish' fear-based society that we are now scared to listen intuitively to what the body needs. After all, we have been so in*doc*trinated to believe that we must take medical drugs for whatever illness that we are now fearful of what may happen if we don't. There are few better motivators than fear, and large sections of the medical drug profession use it well. Remember, anti-obesity drugs are now a multi-billion-dollar industry and one of the most lucrative in the 'medical' field.

This is why it comes as no surprise when some people in the medical profession try to call a programme like this dangerous. Most simply read the front cover and make an instant judgement; others simply aren't willing to accept that the liquid fuel contained within the fibres of nature's purest fruits and vegetables can possible do so much when it comes to *all* illnesses, not just excess weight. They seem to think that almost any period without 'solid food' is harmful for the human body.

In fact, when we are ill the first thing that we go off is our food. This is nature's way of healing; nature's way of saying you cannot deal with the energy-zapping process of trying to digest hard-to-break down food, extract the nutrients and dispose of the wastes. This is why we instinctively crave fruit and water when we are poorly and why the first thing we tend to bring people when they're in hospital is fruit and water.

I hate to see parents who almost force feed their children when they are poorly. Small children will often get a slight temperature and go completely off their food, sometimes for a few days at a time. This again is nature's way of saying, 'Stop the hard-to-digest food and let me heal.' However, we have been so conditioned that we need food at least three to five times a day that parents often override what nature wants and literally push food into their children, even when the child is turning its face away from the food or spitting it out. The parents are clearly doing this out of concern, but sometimes we just need to trust in nature and believe in the power of fruit and vegetables and the body's ability to heal *itself* naturally.

> '*The work of the doctor will, in the future, be ever more that of an educator, and ever less that of a man who treats ailments.*'
> **Lord Horder of Ashcroft**

Luckily, we have a new, more enlightened breed of doctor that is much more willing to look at a more natural approach where possible. I am even recommended by a few doctors, although a depressing majority don't seem to understand how food, or too much of the wrong kind, is responsible for more illness and deaths than all the drugs on the planet *combined*. Many doctors are so blinded by their six years of training with a background of a drug-based therapy that they are unable to see how a person can possibly have all their nutritional needs met through this programme. Indeed, this is yet another thing I get hammered at me, time after time, by some doctors and dieticians: 'I can see how a vegetable-based freshly extracted juice could be of some benefit but ...'

5

Where Will They Get Their Nutrients?

It's funny how doctors, dieticians and, to be fair, many of the people who go on this programme all of a sudden become paranoid about where they are going to get their RDA (Recommended Daily Allowance) of protein, fats, carbohydrates, vitamins, minerals and fibre. When they were eating and drinking junk they weren't overly worried, yet put them on a programme that consists of nothing but fruit, veg and super food supplements, plenty of water and some exercise and suddenly they are worried about whether their body is getting what it requires to function properly!

Why on Earth do people worry about stuff like protein and calcium when they start to consume only fruits and vegetables? It's simple. Ever since we were born we have been bombarded with the 'must have meat and milk for good health' propaganda. We have been so brainwashed on this front that we now believe that it would be dangerous if we didn't – even for a week. We believe we would have a major calcium and protein deficiency. Excuse my language, but there is only one word in the English dictionary that can some up what I need to say right now:

BULLSHIT

All fruits and vegetables contain both calcium and amino acids (the building blocks to protein) in just the ratio we need. In fact, onions and turnips are loaded with calcium; almonds contain almost as much protein as red meat and 6% more calcium per 100g than plain yoghurt. Spirulina – a super food supplement contained in many of the juices on this programme – is the highest natural protein food on the planet with *all* of the essential amino acids required for optimum health. It's also worth pointing out that the largest land animal in the world, with the biggest teeth and some mean muscles, is a bull elephant; and it's an animal which is a vegan – consuming no meat or dairy whatsoever.

The fear of us wasting away and becoming deficient in certain essential nutrients if we don't have a steak with cheese on top solely derives from massive propaganda over the years by the meat and dairy industries.

Steve Arlin, author or *Raw Power*, has been a raw vegan for years yet has a body akin to that of Arnold Schwarzenegger. He eats *only* fruits, seeds, nuts and vegetables – that's it.

Now don't panic, I'm not suggesting you eat nothing but raw food after the 7-day programme, nor am I suggesting you become a vegetarian or vegan. You will see that the Phase 2 Turbo-Charge and Phase 3 Juicy Lifestyle plans are a very 'real' approach to health for all and you will also see that there's some natural 'live' yoghurt included in the 7-day programme. But no, I'm not trying to twist your arm in order to persuade you to dump meat and dairy for life. I'm simply pointing out yet again that you are not going to be nutrient deficient on this programme.

As for fibre, which appears to be the argument about any kind of juice-*only* programme, I want to put your mind at rest. As you will see, and anyone in the medical profession who cares to look at this programme properly will understand, although much of the fibre is removed when you juice, the soluble fibre remains in the juice itself. I have also added psyllium husks, which are a great natural source of dietary fibre, designed to keep you moving – so to speak (*see* Psyllium Husks, page 221). As well as the psyllium husks, many of the smoothies contain whole avocado – probably the most complete food on the planet, with plenty of fibre. I would also like to point out here that fibre *cannot* penetrate through the intestinal wall and it is only the juice contained *within* the fibres of the fruits and vegetables that feeds the body. The fibre is there to act as a 'brush' to keep things moving in the colon, a job which the psyllium husks can do more than adequately.

So on a nutritional front, you really can rest assured that you will have more genuine goodness going into your body during the 7-day programme than the average person has in a month.

When people can find no other argument against the programme they come up with the most common one of them all. Some concede, 'OK, it might be healthy, but if you don't eat solid food for a week ...'

6

Won't You Gain Weight in the Long Run?

Going on this programme does not mean you are guaranteed to pack all the weight back on and more when you start eating again. I know this first hand as I followed a much more drastic juice-only programme than the one you are reading about.

Three-Month Juice Madness

I once went on a 'diet' where I had nothing but freshly extracted juices for three whole months – yes, *nothing* but juice for 12 weeks. It wasn't like this programme where you are having some amazing veggie smoothies and some incredible super foods such as wheatgrass and spirulina. I mean I had *nothing but pure juice*, not even any husks or seeds for added fibre. Was I mad? YES. Would I ever recommend it? NOT IN A MILLION YEARS! Was I uninformed on the juicing front back then? YES. Did I turn orange because of the amount of carrot juice I was having? YES!

However, I only did it out of sheer desperation to rid my body completely of psoriasis. I had had some good results by adding a few juices to what I was normally eating, but I wanted to clear my body completely.

Did I lose weight? YES – big time! And did I lose too much weight? YES. As you can imagine, I lost not only my excess fat, but also my healthy fat and *plenty* of lean muscle tissue too. In fact, my footballer's legs looked like those of a 'heroin chic' model. I would *never, ever* recommend anyone do a juice-only programme for this long.

The reason I bring it up here is not simply to warn against doing a juice-only programme for that long, but to prove that just because you lose weight through liquid only doesn't mean that the minute you stop and return to eating you will end up as big as a house. Yes, I know Oprah Winfrey lost tons of weight when on a liquid-only diet, only to put it all back on and more. It's all about the *quality* of the liquid *together with* how you introduce regular food back into your diet, what you consider to be 'regular food', and how you move your body on a regular basis – which I will cover in depth to make sure your success lasts.

When I started to introduce *good-quality* whole foods back into my diet after my three-month juice-only thing, I soon started to fill out – but I didn't get fat. My muscles returned, I got my legs back, but no double chin was to be seen. In fact, before I started I was overweight, but after eating good food as well as continuing juicing every day, I went to a healthy weight – and have remained there ever since. Again, I wouldn't advocate this, and looking back there was no need for me to do it for so long. The perceived wisdom is that if you go on liquids only you could become obese in the long run because of it.

I'm now a very healthy weight and, like most, if I eat too much and don't exercise I will gain weight. But that's just simple nutritional maths: if I eat too much of the wrong stuff and don't move – I get fat! Call me Mr Obvious but isn't that the same for nearly everyone?

I'll tell you now, if after you do this programme you go back to eating the same amount of rubbish as you did before, guess what? You'll put the weight back on, and the chances are even *more* besides. But again that's got sod all to do with the programme or with Geoffrey Cannon's theory. It's simply because you were gaining weight *before* you went on the programme due to the crap you were eating and drinking and now that you've gone straight back you have picked up where you left off. It amazes me that when people gain weight after a diet they blame the diet. It appears amnesia sets in and they seem to have forgotten the fact they were gaining weight *before* they tried to do something about it and that it's now the diet's fault, not the fact they are eating for their country again and are glued to the sofa. It's not that diets don't work, most of the time it's the person who doesn't work. It never seems to dawn on people that they may have something to do with their own success. If it isn't the diet they blame, you can bet your bottom dollar it will be something else – but not them!

This is why I am covering just about every aspect in order to make sure you continue with Phases 2 and 3, making this a lifestyle change, not just a week's 'diet' to get into your new outfit or whatever.

The truth is I have devised this plan so carefully that you could live on it for three months if you chose – there's no need to and I DON'T advise it, but on a nutritional level you could. This is why I just cannot understand why oh why some doctors and dieticians regard the 7-day plan as dangerous, especially when you can see and feel the results. Sometimes I think we have to just accept that nature is bigger than us. We have to accept that sometimes all of the medical or dietetic training in the world cannot fully explain how the body heals with the power of the liquid contained within fruits and vegetables. You cannot argue with results, and when you stop the junk, flush the body and furnish it with pure juice, amazing things happen. Sometimes we just have to accept that we may not know how it works, but as long as it works – who cares?

There are many examples of how the human body survives, often baffling the medical profession. One such example will help to reiterate a few of my points. If the medical profession thought me living on nothing but juice for three months was mad, then it's positively sane compared to …

7

The David Blaine Diet

David Blaine went for 44 days on *nothing* but water whilst living in a glass box hoisted above Tower Bridge in London. Many people don't believe he actually did this and that somehow it was all an illusion. However, as well as being a remarkable illusionist, David Blaine is also able to demonstrate the most amazing examples of what human beings are capable of. He will push himself over and over again simply to test human endurance. As well as living on nothing but water for 44 days, he has also buried himself alive for 7 days, lived in a block of ice for 3 days, and stood on top of an 80 ft pole for 34 hours before leaping down onto some cardboard boxes. The pole business may not sound like much to everyone, but it is not something that could be achieved in a day. Blaine practised and practised for over a year before getting on that pole. He first stood on a 20ft high pole and learnt from some of the top Hollywood stuntmen how to fall without injury. When he was comfortable with that he went up to 40ft and worked his way to 80ft, never once using a safety net. He also climbed mountains *daily* on a bike in order to make sure that his legs had the strength to stand in one position for 34 hours. He learnt how to fast for long periods and had no food or water for the entire time he was on the pole. So why did he do it? He was afraid of heights and wanted to release himself from that fear. David Blaine is a truly amazing example of what's possible when you *fully* prepare and are *fully* focused.

But what has any of this got to do with this 7lbs in 7 Days Super Juice Plan? Well, it's to provide a little perspective and to once again question the advice of many dieticians, nutritionists and doctors. If this man can go for 44 days stuck in a box with just water, come out alive and return to a normal weight in no time afterwards, then we really do have to ask how any doctor, dietician or nutritionist can possibly say that living on freshly extracted juice for just 7 days is in any way bad for the average overweight and lethargic person. You have to question it even more once you consider that as well as the freshly extracted juice and good-quality supplements, the programme contains plenty of nature's most wholesome food – avocado. We also have to ask, if David Blaine can do something as extreme as that for 44 days, how hard can it possibly be to live on the finest-quality freshly extracted juice and smoothies for a week?

IT'S *EASY* PEASY
LEMON AND CARROT *SQUEEZY*

Have a serious think about it. If David Blaine declared to the world that he was going to live on nothing but freshly extracted juices for one week, do you think for one second it would make the papers? Do you think a documentary would be made about it? Would people say things like, 'Of course he can go for 7 days on juice only. The man's an illusionist and it's a trick?' Umm, methinks not. Why? Because people would say, '*What's so special about that – anyone can do it.*' And it's true – anyone *can* do it! But what people *can* do and what they *will* do are often two very different things. Most people *can* exercise daily, but most do not. Most people *can* eat well daily, but most do not. Most people *can* take their lives to the next level, but most do not. Most people *can* do small things each day that will move them to a more rewarding and compelling life, but most do not. Most people *can* tell the people close to them every day that they love them, but most do not. In reality, most people *can* actually do anything they put their minds to, but the sad reality is most do not.

What people can do and what they will do are often many worlds apart. The simple truth is you *can* do this 7-day programme, you can find the time, you can stay focused, you can lose 7lbs in 7 days, you can tap into an energy you haven't felt for ages, you can give your body an amazing clean for week, and you can *easily* do Phases 2 and 3. The question is not whether you *can*, but *will* you? *Will* you find the time? *Will* you do what it takes? *Will* you cut out the endless list of excuses people use not to move forward in life? Or will you do what most people do when it comes to truly changing this part of their life, simply talk about it but never do it?

Are You a Thinker or a Doer?

So many people are great at talking about a better lifestyle, better health and a slim, sexy, energy-driven body. They are also good at spending copious amounts of time 'reading' tabloid magazines that slag off celebs who happen not to be 100% perfect. They sit around day after day, night after night telling people about the things they are *going* to do, but very few are actively doing anything. Yes, we're all good at *starting* different 'life-changing' programmes, but so few of us see them through or get to the stage where we begin to see, feel and live the results.

I know many people who have read just about every weight loss/health/nutrition book on the planet, yet are still overweight and incredible unhealthy. That's because all of the self-help books, CDs, DVDs and the like mean absolutely nothing without YOU taking action. *The Oxford English Dictionary*'s definition of **Action** is, '**The process of doing something**' – not the process of *thinking* about doing something, but the process of *actually* doing something.

One of the top people from the Toyota corporation was giving a presentation in which he appeared to be giving away some critical information. The audience was amazed at how freely he was willing to share so much information with so many. When asked about his willingness to be so candid, he replied: 'Everyone can listen, but few will act.'

A truer statement has never been made.

There is a great line in the film *Pirates of the Caribbean* where the Commodore says to the character played by Johnny Depp, Jack Sparrow, 'You are without question the worst pirate I've ever heard of,' to which Jack Sparrow replies, 'Yes, but you have heard of me.'

Like him or loathe him, the fact is that we have only heard of David Blaine because of his ability to act, his ability to go from just thinking to actually doing. Your ability to act on this programme (or not to act) will be the difference between this book being a few bits of paper with ink on or a life- and body-changing experience.

The ability to act and see something through is one of the most rewarding things you can do in life. It gives you a sense of fulfilment, achievement, success and is one of the most common pieces of feedback I get from those who do this programme. People feel amazing not only because they have cleaned the system, lost weight and have more energy, but because they made a decision and for once actually followed it through no matter what.

What **Distinguishes** a Successful Person from Others Is Not Their **Strength,** Not Their **Knowledge,** But Rather Their **Will**

The 'Will you or won't you do whatever it takes to do the programme and make this a catalyst for life?' question pretty much comes down to just one thing.

I can honestly say that after being in this business for many years and seeing hundreds of thousands of people from all parts of the globe on this subject, I have concluded that there is just one thing, or one condition if you will, more than any other that prevents people from doing a programme of this nature. It's a condition that seems to be spreading faster than any other and it's one which creates more illness, obesity and unfulfilment than anything else. You may not have heard of its official term but you will know plenty of people with it and you will have suffered from it many times yourself in the past. It is the condition known as ...

8

CBAS
(Can't Be Arsed Syndrome!)

Or, if we are being more politically correct, Can't Be Bothered Syndrome.

And that's the bottom line, isn't it? *Can* you do the programme is a clear 'yes'. Can you be bothered is another question altogether.

EXCUSES, *EXCUSES*, EXCUSES

Can't Be Arsed Syndrome is the antithesis of the ability to take action. It's what *thinkers* suffer from most of the time. It's the one thing – more than anything else – that prevents people from getting from where they are to where they would LOVE to be.

CBAS is a mental attitude and is without question the most destructive mental attitude a person can have. It causes more feelings of failure and unfulfilment than any other.

If you can't be arsed then you won't be reading this sentence. If you can't be arsed and really don't want to do something about your situation, there is no way you would have got this far into the book. In fact, over 90% of people who buy a book of this sort don't even read past the first two chapters. They may have gone from *thinking* about buying a book to actually buying it, but that isn't *real* action. Anyone can buy a book – you don't even have to leave your house these days to accomplish that. So many people think that by the simple act of buying a self-help book they have helped themselves. But it's called a *self-help book* because *you have to help yourself*. The bottom line is that it's up to you. I know any number of people who have books, DVDs and CD courses that have barely been looked at, let alone acted upon – but, hey, they look good in the house and give the impression you are at least *thinking* about life change. You can lead a horse to water and all that. The ability to take action is the key, and as long as you suffer from CBAS you will never take action and never have the body and health you crave.

This is why I know that you personally can be bothered. You have not only got hold of a copy of this book but you are actually reading it. And that is way, way further than most people get. However, the reason I'm sitting here banging away on my keyboard is not just to get you to read the book; it's to get you to take massive action on it so you get the results. Many people buy a book of this sort, but few actually read it and even fewer *act* on it from start *and* finish.

We are all increasingly health conscious these days and we constantly hear people spouting off about how 'Health is the most important thing' and 'If you haven't got your health you've got nothing.' That's all fine and dandy but nine times out of ten they are saying it just before they shove yet another cream bun down their gullet!

Talking good health and *doing* good health are two completely different things. What we 'think' we are doing is often a far cry from what we are actually doing. Talking about doing this programme and actually doing this programme are also two very different things. I know I keep repeating this point, but bizarre as it may sound I actually care about the results you have and you will only achieve results if you take action. And you will only take action if you kick the CBAS and decide once and for all ...

9

No More Excuses!

Over the years I think I've heard them all. In my last book I called this 'The But Syndrome'. *But* I can't because I don't have the time; *But* I can't because I have children; *But* I can't because I'm too old; *But* I can't because it's different for me, etc., etc. I pointed out at the time:

The More **Buts** You Have
the **B i g g e r** **Butt** You Will Have

I think it's safe to say that many people reading this book will want to change their butt, as well as their health and energy levels. However, the only way to change your butt is if you change your but. What I mean by that is changing from your almost automatic '*but* I can't because ...' set of excuses. These are the excuses we use in an attempt to try and justify what is essentially a clear dose of Can't Be Arsed Syndrome.

Everybody can, if they choose, come up with a 'but I can't because ...' for just about anything *and* easily convince themselves and others that it's a perfectly reasonable 'but'. And if you're from the nicer side of town don't think the word 'however' gets you off the hook either!

Instead of automatically saying, '*but* I can't because ...' you should immediately change it to, '*but* if I could what would I need to do in order to make it happen?' By asking yourself a question like that your brain automatically assumes that it *is* actually possible and just needs to spend a short while thinking about it to find an answer. The change of 'but' will then inevitably have a knock-on effect that changes your 'butt'. Conversely, if you say, '*but* I can't because ...' there is simply no way your mind will even attempt to look for a solution and your 'butt' will remain the same.

Most people come up with a set of 'buts' in order not to do a programme of this nature at all. Others will start, but at the first sign of them having to make *any* degree of effort out comes the '*but* I can't because ...' set of excuses.

When testing this programme on a focus group, I asked a few of my friends to try it at the same time. I gave some of them the simple mental preparation (which you will be getting in the next chapter) and two friends no mental preparation whatsoever. All the two friends had were a few A4 sheets of paper with the step-by-step programme on it. I knew that without at least some amount of mental preparation a few 'buts' would rear their ugly heads and that my friends might find it a bit trickier than the others, but I didn't realize to what extent.

Although they started well – as in 'Yes, we are going to do this' and making all the right noises and getting all the right stuff – it didn't take long before the 'buts' kicked in.

One of them, Martin, only got to day 2 before his particular 'but' caused him to cave in. It turned out he didn't just have one 'but' – he had a bucket full of them. 'But it wasn't the right time', 'But I had too much on', 'But I was just so hungry', and this was on just DAY 2! None of these excuses held any water. He said, 'But I had too much on and it wasn't the right time'. You tell me who doesn't have a lot on? And at the same time you tell me about any 7-day period where 'stuff' doesn't happen where it appears 'this is the wrong time to be doing this'? Life has a habit of challenging us, and this is good: it's the very stuff which tests our strength of character and makes us grow as people. However, most people see it as a time to sabotage, a time to 'but' their way to yet another failure. Martin also used the 'But I was just so hungry' excuse and said, 'I just HAD to eat something.' Again I must stress he was only on day 2! Or, to put it another way, he had gone just *one night* without solid food. He wasn't physically hungry at all – he can't have been – he was, after all, getting more genuine nutrition than he had been getting for months. The reality was he had a *mental* hunger, not a physical one. He was feeling mentally deprived, and had a bit of an internal mental tantrum which resulted in the inevitable string of 'buts'.

The same thing happened with the other friend who 'attempted' the programme. His 'buts' were different, but the reason or 'excuses' and the end result were inevitably the same. He lasted one more day than Martin, but that's still only two and a bit days – hardly stretching yourself, I'm sure you'll agree. Now this friend would never, ever like to admit he has failed at anything. He is a strong person who when he sets his mind to something usually achieves it. So his 'but' wasn't 'but I was too busy' or 'but I had too much on' as he knew that wouldn't wash with me. I have already explained how sometimes doctors and dieticians question the programme in terms of nutrition. Unfortunately, we now live in a world where we have such fears about not getting enough of this or that in our diet that it's all too easy to use this as a 'but' excuse.

The man in question exercises quite a lot and decided during the programme to do some calculations. He had worked out that most days his calorie intake on the programme was 1,000 calories. I don't know how he worked that out, especially when one small avocado alone contains 275 calories, but, hey, let's go with it anyway. He reckoned he was exercising daily to the point where he was burning off 400 calories a day. He did the maths (or math if you're from the US!) and came to the conclusion that he was only having 600 calories a day and therefore it was unhealthy – so he caved in.

The reality was that he caved in not because of any genuine lack of calories he was or wasn't having, but for the same reason as Martin – *mental* deprivation. He knew he could have increased his intake of juices and smoothies to meet whatever calorie deficit he perceived he required. I even encourage this as you should always get nutrition if you are *genuinely* hungry. So why didn't he? Because he had a 'Sod It' moment, suffered from an instant dose of CBAS and came up with a suitable 'but' to justify his action not only to other people (namely me!) but also to himself. That sounds harsh, but most people skirt around the issue, which makes me immediately think of the famous lines from the film *A Few Good Men*:

'Do you want the **truth*!'**
'You can't **handle** *the* **truth.*'**

The fact is most people can't handle the truth. Especially when the truth is most people try to justify their CBAS excuses as genuine reasons.

The reality is that there are more than enough calories to sustain the average person, so even with some high-impact exercising every day, you won't collapse. I know this personally because when I did the 7-day programme I ran a half marathon on day 5 as well as working out for at least an hour a day on the other 6 days.

I'm not saying this to impress you, but to impress *upon* you that you are not about to waste away on this programme. The 'dip' in energy that my friend felt was simply due to the withdrawal from drug-like foods and drinks such as white refined sugar and caffeine. It was *not* caused by a calorie deficiency. In fact, most of the time the symptoms of physical withdrawal people think they get from coming off certain 'foods' and 'drinks' are often extremely mild. Nine times out of ten they aren't actually physically deflated, but *mentally* deflated. They are once again feeling mentally deprived and so the tantrum rears its head – and once again the set of 'buts' arrives on the scene.

I'm far from the only one who has managed to exercise to a high intensity during this juice-only programme. I know a girl who also ran a half marathon on day 6, another person who did the back-breaking work of 'mucking out' horses for 2 hours a day *and* doing 45 minutes of mini-trampolining, and many, many, many more who either did loads of yoga, weight-training, swimming, walking and so on. Most of the juices have celery, cucumber and apple in them, all of which add up to nature's finest balance of sodium and potassium – minerals which we lose when working out. These juices not only replenish our stores but also help with any aches, pains and cramps usually associated with exercise. So the whole 'but I'm not getting enough calories' excuse really is flawed.

What is a calorie anyway?

We hear about calories all the time, but ask most people what a calorie actually is and you will see a blank face. A calorie is the amount of energy (heat) needed to raise one gram of water by one degree centigrade. Confused? Me too.

Calories are a misguided measurement of what or how much of what we should eat. For example, Antony Worrall Thompson (a famous chef in the UK) created a recipe which was considered so unhealthy that it even had newspaper headlines such as, '**Is This the Unhealthiest Recipe Ever?**' and '**Worrall Thompson's Snickers Pie Condemned as a Health Hazard**'. According to the Food Commission's calculations, a *single* serving of the pie contains 22 teaspoons of fat, 11 teaspoons of sugar and has 1,250 calories – not that surprising when you consider the pie contains 5 Snickers bars! Now, if we go by calories then the average man or woman would only need to consume 1½–2 slices of the pie each day to meet their body's needs. But even if you know nothing about food, nutrition and calories, does that make any sense to you? Does anyone honestly believe that on a nutritional or calorific level two slices of Worrall's Snickers Pie would meet anyone's needs? If we go by my friend's reason (excuse) for quitting, then I can only assume that if I had put him on a diet of Snickers Pie he would have thought it a much safer bet for his health and energy levels than the 'live' juices and smoothies on this programme.

In reality, *nutritional* needs and *calorific* needs are completely different. According to 'calorie experts' the simple act of pushing your finger on the button of a remote control uses 1 calorie. So, by that theory, if you changed channel on your TV 400–500 times you would burn as many calories as if you ran on a treadmill at a fairly high intensity for 1 hour. I think we all agree that is total RUBBISH! Let's also not forget that on the Atkins diet people could eat as many calories as they liked in the form of fat and protein, yet still lose weight – and they didn't exercise. We now know that the Atkins diet had several flaws, but I'm only using it here to demonstrate that calories mean nothing when it comes to optimum health.

Do you actually know how many calories you have each day? I don't know about you but I haven't got a clue and I don't care – I feel bloody good and I'm not wasting away. Some days I eat very little and others I have a mother of an appetite, but so what? I eat according to whether I'm genuinely hungry or not; not because it happens to be 6 p.m. or because I'm caught up in this 'Oh I must have so many calories a day' nonsense.

If my friend had not been *consciously* aware of what he had been taught about calories, he would have been fine. However, he was caught up in the *belief* that what he was having couldn't sustain him, and belief can be stronger than oak.

In the same way that placebos can help and have been shown in some cases to 'cure' disease, the converse belief that something cannot work can be just as strong. Just the belief that you will get weak if you *think* you're not getting enough calories can be enough to cause you to actually feel weak.

BUT, *NOTHING!*

This programme is not only nutritionally sound but *also* calorie sound: the two are not the same. The programme is also based on nature's principles of what calories your body requires and not what we have been conditioned to believe. What you may think you need and what your body actually needs are often a world apart.

One of my friends used calories as an excuse and the other used 'I had a lot on', but I know that no matter what is going on in your life you can, if you stop the negative buts, easily complete the programme.

Like so many others, I have a busy schedule at the best of times and the first week I did this programme was no exception. I had to leave my house one morning at 6 a.m. and didn't return until 11 p.m. I had meetings all day and even had to 'do' lunch and dinner with some of the top people from a major worldwide company. Despite this I still kept to the programme and had *nothing* but juices. All it took was a little preparation on the mental and physical front. I made sure I woke up early, made my juices for the whole day, stored them in flasks and off I went. Was it ideal? NO. Was it the best available? YES! Were some of the nutrients lost throughout the day? YES. How did I go to lunch and dinner and not feel uncomfortable about not eating? EASY, I just told them what I was doing and that there would always be an 'exception' during any 7-day period, so please respect my decision. You will be amazed at just how much people respect anyone who makes a decision and sees it through, especially top people of worldwide companies.

I have said that the only way to change your 'butt' is to change your 'buts'. Instead of '*but* I can't because ...', simply change to, '*but* if I could, what would I need to do to make it happen?' Instead of me just saying, 'But I can't as I have to be out all day and do lunch and dinner', I changed my but and asked, 'But what would I need to do in order to make sure I could work around it?' As soon as I asked the question my brain came up with the answers. Get up early, make sure you have big enough flasks, drink plenty of water and make sure you explain the situation to the people who you are going to lunch and dinner with in *advance*. I also had to do a family lunch on the Sunday (day 7). Once again I explained *in advance* what I was doing. The question is not whether a 'special' situation will occur during the 7 days, but what you will do *when* it occurs.

There are no *reasons* why people can't do this, just *excuses*. There is also no reason on the planet why you can't find it easy. There are always two ways to skin a cat, as they say, and there are always two ways to go about a programme like this. One is the way my two friends went about it – the hard way; the other way therefore is clearly ...

10

The Easy Way

I have said it from the start of this book – and I mention it in all of my books: The single most important aspect of this programme is the right psychology, the right way of thinking. If you go into this programme without extremely good mental preparation, you may succeed through sheer grit, willpower and determination, but you won't make it easy for yourself. It's more than likely, though, that you won't reach the end, and before you know where you are you'll be back eating and drinking the same old rubbish. This is not what you want and it's not what I want for you either.

What is crazy is that there is no reason on the planet why anyone should find the programme hard. I'm not saying that some people don't find it hard – as you saw with my two friends, some clearly do – but what I am saying is there is no *need* to. The reality is that if you do struggle it will *only* be because of what *you* say to yourself.

That's it and that's all. I wish it were more complicated, but the bottom line is, if you sit and whinge about what you think you can't have you will find it hard, and if you don't do that you won't! It really is as simple as that.

When I say 'what you *think* you can't have', the reality is you *can* have what the blooming hell you like. After all, *you* are the one who is choosing to do this because *you* want to clean your system and *you* want the mental and physical rewards that come with it. It won't make any difference to me, the people up the road or anyone else for that matter. *You* want to do this because *you* want to look and feel bloody good.

This is what people forget when they change their eating and lifestyle – *they* are choosing to do it. This is why it makes absolutely no sense at all to go into what is essentially a self-imposed mental tantrum. And isn't that pretty much all it comes down to?

The Power of CAN'T

Words are far more powerful that any 'physical' withdrawal from drug-like foods and drinks. In fact, even with a drug like nicotine, which has been described by some experts as 'just as hard to give up as heroin', the 'suffering' people experience when stopping is caused primarily by *words*, not the nicotine. The most powerful of all words when it comes to changing what you eat or when on a detox like this is the word CAN'T. I have a great acronym for it:

Constant And Never-ending Tantrum

It's this simple:

If you say 'I want but I *can't* have' – you will suffer.

If you say 'I *can* but I don't want to have' – you won't.

By removing the 'T' from 'CANT' you have effectively removed the *self-imposed* tantrum. Let me give you an example.

One of the people who was in the focus group called me up on day 4 and said, 'Jay, help, I want some chocolate and it's driving me crazy that I can't have any. What can you do?' Straight away you can hear that it's clearly a *mental* craving as the body never craves chocolate. I now hear screams of 'ARE YOU KIDDING ME, VALE!', but seriously, it's the mind that craves chocolate, not the body. As it was a false mental need and not a genuine physical one it was up to her, and not me, to get rid of the 'craving'. A mental 'craving' is simply a self-imposed mental tantrum and if the tantrum stops the craving does too. With that in mind I simply said that she should go to the shop, buy some chocolate, eat it and call me when she got back. I then said goodbye and hung up. The phone rang again almost immediately and the woman said, 'WHAT? Did you just say I should go to the shop and buy some chocolate and eat it – are you kidding?'

'No!'

'Hang on. Let me get this right. I'm on *your* 7 lbs in 7 Days juice programme. You're the guy who's into healthy eating and the person who even wrote a book called *Chocolate Busters*. And here you are telling me to go and eat some chocolate. That's not the sort of help I expected!'

'Look, if you called me and said you want a banana I would have told you to go and have one. Instead you said you wanted to have some chocolate so I told you to go and have some. What's wrong with that?'

'The reason I'm phoning you is because I DON'T WANT TO HAVE ANY CHOCOLATE – I WANT TO COMPLETE THIS PROGRAMME' ... and, yes, she was shouting a lot by this stage!

'Oh,' I said, 'so you *don't* want any chocolate. Thank God for that. So how are you?'

There was then a little silence before she said, 'Don't try to get clever.' But I wasn't trying to get clever. I was trying to point out that what she had was a self-imposed tantrum caused only by what *she* was saying to herself. Effectively she was moping around for something which she hoped she wouldn't have. How crackers is that – moping around for something which you hope you won't have? Imagine a child kicking up a fuss because he didn't have a toy but the minute you offered it he started shouting, saying he didn't actually want it. Imagine if he was feeling deprived without it, but didn't really want to have it – a bit of a no-win situation, I would say. This was precisely the position this woman was in and precisely the position *all* people who struggle put themselves through when changing what they eat or stopping smoking. The cause of her problem was not some genuine chocolate deficiency, but rather a feeling of mental deprivation. The way to remove it is extremely simple. This was my reply to her,

> **'Please** *don't take this the wrong way, but the only way to solve your* **problem** *is this: either have the chocolate and shut up, or don't have it and shut up, but whatever you do,*
> **SHUT UP!'**

Although taken aback a little at first, she soon realized what I was saying was true. She didn't actually want the chocolate, which is why she phoned. What she wanted was to complete the programme and have the tremendous mental and physical results which come from it. And this is precisely what you want too. It is why you have read this far into the book. If you dump the excuses and don't mope around for things you actually don't want to have anyway, then it's easy. If you come up with a bunch of 'buts', start to bitch and feel sorry for yourself, then of course you will find it hard. It's not rocket science when you look at it.

Should I Say Anything or Just Bite My Tongue?

Prime examples of just what can happen if not armed with the correct way of thinking are my two friends I mentioned earlier. I have told you about Martin, the friend who only managed to 'survive' for two days before 'butting' his way to defeat, but what I didn't tell you was the full story of what happened to him.

During the early evening of day 2 he experienced what I now refer to as a 'Bread Head'. This is where he had such a *mental* craving for bread (in this case) that when he went to take a bite he bit so quickly and so hard that he literally bit a hole in his tongue (if you ever see the *7 lbs in 7 Days* DVD you will see exactly what I mean). The tongue is an organ that repairs itself perhaps faster than any other and yet even when he woke up the following morning the hole still hadn't healed. He ended up having to go to hospital where he had two stitches! If he had only said the right things to himself he would never have had to bite his tongue.

Clearly this is an *extremely* rare case, even for those people who have no mental prep. What I want you to get from this tale is that he wasn't suffering physically *before* he took a chuck of bread; he simply had a mother of a *mental* craving. The point is he had a bread *head*, not a bread stomach. In exactly the same way, the woman who called me had a choc head rather than a choc stomach.

I am pleased to say that after my conversation with the 'choc head' woman, she was fine and not only completed the 7-day programme but also the Phase 2 Turbo-Charge plan as well and dropped 19lbs in all. The irony is that if she had shut up and had actually had some she wouldn't have been *able* to shut up. What I mean is she would have immediately felt like a failure and it would have driven her mad. By shutting up and not having some, she went on to succeed.

Diet Mentality

This is why at the start of this book I mentioned that this approach isn't a diet approach. Dieting is a mentality. If you feel deprived and are constantly looking at others with envy then you are *on a diet*; if you don't feel deprived then you aren't!

It is the feeling of deprivation that creates a diet mentality. I know people who as soon as they start a 'diet' immediately start to feel like they are on a diet. This can be as soon as the first morning, even if they are the kind of person who didn't usually eat breakfast. The minute they wake up they are conscious that they are on a 'diet', focus on what they can't have and immediately enter the world of diet mentality. There is no need whatsoever to spiral into this approach. As long as you don't suffer from CANT, you

won't have a problem and you won't constantly feel like
you are on a diet. You will be aware that you are on Phase
1 of *changing your diet*, not going *on a diet*.

A World of Abundance Yet an Attitude of Lack

Another key mental tool which again appears obvious and
easy yet is seldom practised is that of gratitude. In the West
we live in a world of abundance, yet most people focus on
what they haven't got, as opposed to feeling grateful for
what is available to them. In fact, it appears the more we
have the more *unfulfilled* we feel. If you feel unfulfilled you
inevitably feel empty. People try to fill the empty feeling
with all sorts of stuff from food to shopping. It's all about
the instant 'hit', the instant fix of fulfilment. The only
problem with this is that true fulfilment is rarely achieved
and an almost permanent feeling of emptiness is
experienced.

An 'attitude of gratitude' will make such a difference to
you on this programme. It moves you from the 'I can't
have' child-like mental tantrum to one of empowerment
and fulfilment. As we speak there are people around the
world walking 20 miles a day to get water, and over half
the world's population lives on less than 50p a day. If you
have a roof over your head, food for the next week, pretty

good health and clean running water available to you for washing and drinking, you are in the top 8% of the population of the world. Yet most people complain that they are not in the top 2%. Is this a guilt trip way of looking at things? NO. Is it a way of saying, 'Stop bloody moaning'? YES! Is it time for some perspective? Again YES.

The truth is we all need perspective and whether I use David Blaine or the millions of people around the world who would give their right arm to be where you are today is unimportant. I only have two objectives in writing this book, to get people to read it and then do it.

You have an opportunity that most in the world can only dream of. For you it's not even a case of whether the food is available, it's whether you are going to moan and suffer from CBAS.

Make Life a **'Get to'**, Not a **'Have to'**.

Remember that you don't HAVE to do this programme, you WANT to do it; you have the opportunity to GET to do it. There is a big difference between 'having to' and 'getting to'. Even when you say it, don't you just feel different? If you say, 'I *have* to go out tonight,' doesn't it feel so different to when you say, 'I *get* to go out tonight'?

During the next 7 days you will get the chance to furnish your system with fine liquid nutrition, the chance to clean your body of any toxins and pollution, the chance to get the body you want, to test your character, to grow as a human, to expand your world, to challenge yourself, a chance to take time out from the 'I don't have what I want' feeling-sorry-for-yourself world to one where you can feel grateful.

As corny as it sounds, life isn't about just getting through, it's about the journey. The same goes for this programme. You don't just want to 'hang on in there' for a week. You want to have a life too. You don't have to sit in like a hermit; there's nothing stopping you from going out and living during this time. All you are doing is not eating solid food for a week, but it's not as if you're not being fed. In fact, you will probably be fed more during this programme than you have been in years. After a few days you'll have more energy and time than you've had for ages.

When I first did the 7-day plan I went to lunches, dinners, parties and even ran half a marathon – it wasn't hard. Trying to walk with no shoes in blistering heat for many miles with no water in search of food and shelter is hard – this isn't. You are doing this to change your life and to feel more fulfilled (and slimmer). There is no faster way on Earth to feel fulfilled than when you live with an attitude of gratitude.

Your Life Is a Direct Result of What *You* Feed Yourself

Your life is shaped by what you feed yourself. I don't just mean what you feed yourself physically: I'm talking about what you feed yourself audibly, spiritually and visually.

Food is just one aspect of health, and what gets beamed into your ears and eyes on a daily basis has a much more profound effect on your mental and physical health than you could ever possibly realize.

The biggest influence on our waistlines and health in general (other than food) is something that has taken over many people's lives almost without them being aware of it. Not only has it taken over their lives, it has *become* their lives. As physical movement plays a part in this programme, and given that the next subject creates more lack of movement than any other, I feel it an extremely important item to include. I can, of course, only be talking about one thing …

11

TV (Total Vegetable)

'Britons watch more TV yet read less than any other country in Europe.'

Of all the gadgets in the world today none will hypnotize you and rob you of huge chunks of your life more than television. The average Briton now watches an unbelievable 4–6 hours of TV a day. Television is now the most used babysitter in the West.

By the time **children** *reach 6 years of age, they will have spent, on average,* **one year** *of their life watching* **TV!**

But it's not just our precious time it sucks from our lives: there are now many reports that show that in some cases watching TV can be just as harmful as the wrong foods and even smoking.

I can almost hear the panic in your voice. 'OK, Jay, one week of nothing but juice, but are you now saying no TV?' The sad reality is that many people would find it easier to do one week with only juices than go without TV. Now, don't panic. I am not suggesting you go TV cold turkey or that you stop watching the amount you are already watching – that's your call. But I do want to share with you some info about TV that hopefully may get you to switch it off and get moving.

TV Can Make You Fat!

Let me be clear about this. I don't mean that while you are watching TV you aren't exercising or moving, so you have a greater chance of gaining weight. I actually mean that just by watching TV you have a greater chance of gaining weight than if you sat and did nothing. Before you throw this book in the bin, thinking I have completely lost the plot, please hear me out.

A study entitled 'Effects of television on metabolic rate: potential implications for childhood obesity' showed that children's and adolescents' metabolic rates were 'significantly lower' when they watched TV than when they weren't doing anything. It turns out that the hypnotic gaze of the 'life in a box' slows down your metabolism! On average, the children and adolescents in the study burned the equivalent of 211 kilocalories *less* per day than if they did diddly squat. The authors of the report concluded:

> 'Television viewing has a fairly profound lowering
> effect of metabolic rate and may be a mechanism for
> the relationship between obesity and amount of
> television viewing.'

And what do we do at the same time as watching TV? Yep – eat. Not only do we eat, but we tend to eat more when watching TV than at almost any other time. According to Dr Aric Sigman, author of the excellent book *Remotely Controlled*, watching television makes children and adults eat more, even if they are not physically hungry. This is borne out by a study entitled 'Television Viewing Nearly Adds an Additional Meal to Daily Intake'. So our metabolism is *slower* at the very time we consume *more* food. Another study showed that people who ate their food to calming music and no TV ate *much* slower and had much less food than those who watched TV while they ate.

TV Can Turn Your Kids Nuts!

Not only can the simple act of watching TV make you fatter than if you sat and did nothing but apparently it can turn your kids nuts too. It seems it is not just sugar and caffeine that can make your kid look like they've just swallowed a bucket of Prozac – it's TV too. In August 1999 a study by the American Academy of Pediatrics (AAP) showed that early TV exposure is associated with problems at age 7 which 'are consistent with a diagnosis of ADHD' (Attention Deficit Hyperactivity Disorder). They concluded that the banning of all TV time during the formative years of brain development 'may reduce children's subsequent risk of developing ADHD'.

There is no question that a combination of junk TV and junk food has a profound effect on children's behaviour and development. There is also no doubt that this same combination has a similar effect on our behaviour and our development as adults. Clearly, getting rid of the junk food and replacing it with the finest juices on Earth will have an incredibly beneficial effect on your body shape and overall health. However, if you get rid of junk TV as well as junk food and replace it with increased physical movement, you will find it has more of an impact on your mental and physical health than you could possibly imagine.

Life = Movement
Movement = *Life*

Without movement there is no life. In fact, if you aren't moving at all you are DEAD! It is no surprise that with such a small amount of physical exercise going on and so much sitting on furniture watching other bits of furniture (TV), so many people do feel, well … dead.

The average person spends less than one hour a week doing physical exercise. I don't mean walking up the stairs or getting up to put a DVD on. I mean *real* exercise – the sort that makes you sweat. At the same time, the average person spends 35–40 hours each week watching TV.

One of the many benefits you will find on this programme is that when you are no longer numbing yourself with 'food' you won't want to 'slump' in front of the TV. You will find, like the vast majority who do this programme, that as your body becomes cleaner and your energy level increases you will actually *want* to exercise more (as unlikely as that may sound to some at this stage).

The Gift of Movement

As with juices we can also use the 'attitude of gratitude' with exercise in order to enhance and enjoy the experience. I am extremely fortunate to have all of my limbs in good working order, but there are many people who don't. I can honestly say that if I ever think I *have* to exercise I soon change my approach so I *get* the opportunity to exercise. I can honestly say that I feel it an insult not to exercise and eat and drink well. It's an insult to have the gift of movement and not use it and it's an insult to have fresh produce available and the opportunity to extract the fine juices from it and not do it. It's even more of an insult not to eat it and then *complain* about eating too much of the other stuff.

When it comes to exercise, again the excuses start, but we can all do something. My motto is simple:

If you can move –
then m*o*v*e!*

I love using my mini-trampoline. It's a soft-bounce trampoline and very different to the usual ones you find. I stock up my MP3 player with a bit of Robbie and I'm bouncing like a mad thing. I also love football, tennis, swimming and just about any game. On the retreats I always introduce some kind of physical activity – it just makes it more fun. I want people to think 'I get to play today' instead of thinking 'I have to exercise'. Remember, when you make life a 'get to' rather than a 'have to', true joy and fulfilment are yours for the taking. You get to enjoy the journey too.

At the 'Intimate' retreat we have group mini-trampolining sessions. It's such an amazing way to get into shape and other than swimming it's the only exercise on the planet that uses every single muscle! Rebounding even has NASA approval:

'Rebound exercise is the most **efficient** *and* **effective** *exercise yet devised by man.'*

But that's my bag – you may choose something completely different. I know loads of people who hated running but now love it. It's amazing what some good music and an attitude of 'running is a wonderful opportunity to have some me time and let my thoughts just run away' can do. They now think running is a *get to* and not a *have to* – and that's the key to whole programme.

I have done all I can do. Now it's your call. You have the opportunity to read the rest of the book and do a programme that could well change more things in your life than just your stomach. I love to hear the feedback, so please let me know how you get on. Whether it's via e-mail, letter or video diary, the juicy team never tire of the inspirational stories. So, until I either read your letter, see you on video or meet you personally at a retreat, I will leave you with some final words. Most people talk a great life, but very few act in order to change. If you are going to do it, then do it – don't talk about it. When I hear people saying, 'I'm *thinking* of doing ...' my eyes just glaze over – it means nothing. But when I here someone saying, 'I'm in the middle of ...' or 'I've started the ...' I'm all ears. On that note I'll leave you with the words of Johann Wolfgang Von Goethe, who puts the whole thing in a nutshell:

'Whatever you **CAN** do,
or dream you can do, begin it.
BOLDNESS has genius,
power and magic in it.
Begin it **NOW**.'

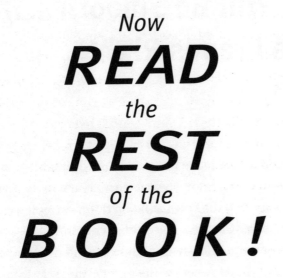

12

All Will Be Smooth ... *if* the Prep Is Right!

Years ago, I used to be, amongst many other things, a painter and decorator. The one part I hated more than any other was filing the holes, sanding down, stripping old wallpaper off the walls and so on; in other words – I hated the preparation. However, if I didn't spend time preparing correctly I would never get the result I was looking for.

The best part of decorating is in the application – watching the paint go on and seeing the transformation from old to new. The worst part is seeing the lumps, bumps and cracks coming through if you *didn't prepare properly*.

The same applies to this programme. The best part is the application –the feeling and seeing the transformation from old to new. And without the right preparation, you simply will not do the programme to the letter and, as with decorating, you'll soon see the lumps and bumps! This 7-day programme requires the right application:

And this will only happen with the right preparation!

'One of the most important rules of Personal Effectiveness is the 10/90 rule.' This statement comes from the excellent book *Eat That Frog* by Brian Tracy:

> *'... the first 10 percent of time that you spend planning and organizing your work, before you begin, will save you as much as 90 percent of the time in getting the job done once you have started.'*

Preparation,
Preparation,
Preparation.

Preparation is without question the key to making this plan as easy as possible. It is also the key to making sure that the 7-day programme becomes a catalyst to a lifelong healthy lifestyle instead of 'yet another diet'. This is why I keep going on about making sure you read the entire book *before* you start as it is incredibly important to have the correct preparation in order to make the programme easy and even enjoyable (as alien as that may sound at this stage).

If, for example, you wake on the first morning of the programme and you have to rush out and shop for everything you need, the chances are you will be overwhelmed and throw in the towel at the first hurdle.

By reading the book, making sure you have everything you need, planning and organizing the week, you will save yourself at least 90% of any stress or hassle you would have had to endure without getting yourself prepared.

So with that in mind I have tried to make life much easier by introducing ...

13

The Juice Master's 7 lbs in 7 Days Super Juice Pack

When testing this programme on myself and others, I asked for as much feedback as possible in order to make the programme as easy as possible. Everyone mentioned that a DVD showing exactly how to make each juice and smoothie, a coaching audio CD to keep motivated, and some kind of wall chart which had all the day-by-day juices and smoothies for easy reference, would be extremely useful. They also mentioned that if there was some kind of pack which contained all of the main supplements in order to save time shopping and hunting, that would also be extremely helpful. So, after listening very carefully to all the feedback, I have put together a '7 lbs in 7 Days Super Juice Pack'.

The pack includes the new motivational *7 lbs in 7 Days* CD; the *7 lbs in 7 Days* DVD (which shows you how to make all of the juices in the programme, gives many juicing tips, how to work and clean a juicing machine, how to make a juice in super-fast time, and it also has some footage of people who have done the programme so you can see the results for yourself *before* you even start); a laminated handy-size 7lbs in 7 Days wall planner (with all the juice/smoothie recipes and the order in which to have the juices); some good-quality wheatgrass, spirulina, some Juice Master's Ultimate Super Food, and a Juice Master Flask – perfect for storing your juices.

The pack not only takes some of the legwork out of getting prepared, but also the CD and DVD are designed to keep you focused, motivated and fully educated so that you actually complete the programme. You will save money too as the items work out much cheaper when in the pack than bought individually. You can then re-use the DVD, CD and wall chart in the future *when* you do the programme again ... and again. I'm also a great believer that if a job's worth doing it's worth doing right; if you get the pack you are sure to give yourself every chance of making sure you do it right.

It's funny how many people will invest huge amounts of money on *external* personal hygiene but will rarely make any sort of investment on their inner sanctuary. The irony of this is that the external appearance is often a direct reflection of what's happening on the inside.

Having said all of that, please remember that the 7lbs in 7 Days Super Juice Programme can still be done without the pack. I have simply put it together as the majority of people who have already done the programme have asked for all or various aspects of it. I want to make this as easy for you as possible and, in today's busy world, I know that if you can just pick up the phone or have a click on your mouse and get everything you need, it's one less thing to have to think about. If you have the book, the pack, a juicer and a blender you're good to go!

However, whether you get the pack or not, here is a full and comprehensive list of everything you will need for the next seven days and beyond ...

14

All the Juicy Stuff You Will Need for the Programme

➤ **A juice extractor.** I get juicers sent to me from all over the world and I must say I have received my fair share of rubbish. Whenever I put my name to a product I always like to make sure that it is good value. At one time this was out of my hands and a juicer with my name on it hit the shelves – it didn't help my reputation. The good news is that I'm now in *full* and total control of which juicers and smoothie makers have my endorsement. There are a few different types of juicer (*see* Which Juicer? page 207) and I recommend just a couple that can do the job.

➤ **A good blender/smoothie maker** (*see* Which Blender/Smoothie Maker?, page 212).

➤ **Wheatgrass.** You will either need a wheatgrass juicer and a tray of ready-grown wheatgrass, wheatgrass powder, ready juiced wheatgrass, or a Juice Master Wheat Grass Kit™. There are several ways to get the goodness of this super food into the programme. (*See* pages 217–21 or **www.juicemaster.com**.)

➤ **The *7 lbs in 7 Days* CD.** This can be bought separately and is a very good mental tool to help with the programme. Clearly this is optional. (*See* 'The Power of a Coach', page 199.)

➤ **Juice Master's Ultimate Super Food.** I wish to make clear here that all the supplements are OPTIONAL. JM's Ultimate Super Food is exactly that – dried food. It is *not a* vitamin or mineral pill, but rather a combination of natural food ingredients, which also happen to be loaded with antioxidants, vitamins and minerals. You can clearly do the programme without it, but as I am unsure as to the quality of the fruits and vegetables you will be using, I fully recommend it as part of the programme and beyond. In addition to what the programme says, you are free to mix with some water and drink throughout the day. This gives you two reasons to drink. One to keep hydrated and two to get some good alkalising nutrients into your body during the programme on top of the juices and smoothies. (See **www.juicemaster.com** for details.)

➤ **Good-quality acidophilus bacteria capsules.** *Good-quality* friendly bacteria are again optional but I would highly encourage this one. Most people have an overgrowth of *Candida* in the gut and a great deal of good bacteria has been destroyed. This needs to be replaced and those ubiquitous small bottles of yoghurt are not going to do the trick effectively. Simply get some live acidophilus in capsule form and empty the contents into a juice. It can be purchased in all good health food shops.

➤ **Spirulina.** You can buy this super food from any good health shop or on the website. (*See* Spirulina, page 213.)

➤ **Mini-trampoline.** If you are going to get a mini-trampoline it's worth investing in a really good one. There are several models I recommend but be careful of cheap 'rebounders' as they can 'jar' your joints and have the opposite effect of what you are looking for. At our retreats we always use a mini-trampoline as part of the programme and I cannot recommend this form of fun exercise enough. I am almost as passionate about rebounding as I am juicing. See website for recommendations.

➤ **A portable music player.** Clearly this is optional, but there is no question that you will always do that little bit more when a good track comes on. Personally, I would do about half or less of the exercise I do without the power of good music. Any MP3 player is worth the investment – the iPod being the most famous, but there are other great ones on the market.

➤ **A good flask.** One of the main problems with flasks is the smell and 'taint' that tends to be left after storing juice for a while, no matter much you clean them. This is why I have put the Juice Master stamp of approval on Sigg flasks, which have a hygienically coated interior to avoid tainting. See www.juicemaster.com for a Juice Master branded Sigg Flask.

➤ **Fruit & veg.** See opposite for the full shopping list …

7lbs in 7 Days Shopping List

This can be downloaded free from www.juicemaster.com

Shopping List for Days 1–3

Get the following items the day *before* you start the programme:

➤ A copy of *The Juice Master: Turbo-Charge Your Life in 14 Days.* This is optional, but it is highly recommended, especially if you want to do Phases 2 and 3 effectively. The idea is for you to start reading the book on Days 3/4 and have it finished by Day 7. The book will be extremely valuable not only in terms of the best way forward from the 7 days, but it will also help a great deal while you are still on this first part of the plan in terms of keeping you in the right frame of mind. If you already have this book, please make sure you follow the instructions and re-read it from Days 3–7. The book is available in all good bookshops and on the website.

➤ 2 lemons – wax free if possible

➤ 6 limes

➤ 3 ripe avocados

➤ 35 apples – not Granny Smiths, they just don't juice well

➤ 3 medium pineapples

➤ 2½ cucumbers

➤ 5 carrots

➤ 4 sticks of celery

- ➤ 1 head of broccoli
- ➤ 1 raw beetroot
- ➤ 1 courgette
- ➤ A stem of fresh ginger
- ➤ 200g natural unsweetened organic yoghurt. If you are vegan or complete dairy free you can use soya yoghurt with friendly bacteria.
- ➤ 1–2 trays of freshly grown wheatgrass, wheatgrass powder or Juice Master Ready Juiced Wheatgrass – see **www.juicemaster.com** for all of above.
- ➤ 100g bottle spirulina – this can be found in all good health shops or at **www.juicemaster.com**
- ➤ 1 bottle of Power Greens – this is optional, but if you do buy a bottle it will last you well over a month. See website for details on this.
- ➤ 1 bottle of high-potency probiotic (friendly bacteria) capsules – I recommend either Udo's Super 5s or Super 8s and these can be found in all good health stores or on the website. If you can't get Udo's, there are several other good makes.
- ➤ 1 bag of watercress
- ➤ 1 bag of kale
- ➤ 1 bag of spinach
- ➤ 1 bag of parsley
- ➤ 1 bag of alfalfa sprouts – these can be found in any good health shop
- ➤ 1 bulb of fresh fennel – optional, to make fresh tea
- ➤ A few sprigs of fresh mint – optional, to make fresh tea
- ➤ 3 good pinches of cinnamon

➤ 1 banana
➤ Ice cubes. Clearly you make these but you do need to have plenty ready – veggie juice really does taste soooooo much better when cold!

Shopping List for Days 4–7

➤ 2 lemons – wax free if possible
➤ 4 limes
➤ 2 ripe avocados
➤ 39 apples – not Granny Smiths
➤ 2 Golden Delicious apples
➤ 4 medium/large pineapples
➤ 3 cucumbers
➤ 1 carrot
➤ sticks of celery
➤ A head of broccoli
➤ 1 raw beetroot
➤ 1 courgette
➤ A stem of fresh ginger
➤ 450/500g natural organic yoghurt
➤ 1 small bottle of cinnamon powder
➤ 1 bag of watercress
➤ 1 bag of kale
➤ 1 bag of spinach
➤ 1 bag of parsley
➤ 1 bag of alfalfa sprouts – these can be hard to get, so simply leave out if you can't get them

➤ 1 bulb of fresh fennel – optional, to make fresh tea
➤ A few sprigs of fresh mint – optional, to make fresh tea.

Phase 1

The 7 lbs in 7 Days Plan

DAY 1

To get your stomach fired up I highly recommend waking
up each morning of the programme to some hot water
with lemon. Simply get a slice of wax-free lemon, put in
mug and pour over some hot water. You are welcome to
drink as many of these as you like each day. At night I
would recommend changing to hot water with fresh fennel
or fennel teabags.

Juices 'n' Smoothies

7 a.m. (......)   **Hot water (with lemon, lime** or **mint)**

8 a.m. (......)   **JM's Super Juice** (*see* page 142)

11 a.m. (......)   **JM's Super Juice**

2 p.m. (......)   **JM's Super Chute Juice** (*see* page 146)

5 p.m. (......)   **JM's Turbo Express** (*see* page 148)

8 p.m. (......)   **JM's Lemon/Ginger Zinger** (*see* page 158)

9 p.m. (......)   **Fennel** or **mint tea** or **JM's Hot 'n' Spicy**
                   (*see* page 150)

(NOTE: Since the times I have set out in the plan might not exactly fit
in with your plans and lifestyle, please fill in your own meal and
break times in the spaces provided.)

Juicy Exercise for Day 1

Morning: 1 x 20/30-minute workout

Early Evening: 1 x 20/30-minute workout

Juicy Comments for Day 1

Drink your juice slowly! This is for the whole programme. Always 'chew' your juices in the mouth to allow for the enzymes in your saliva to act with the food. It also gives time for a signal to be sent to your stomach telling it to get ready for food.

Initially, some people feel tired on the programme, although many don't. For those who do it is often because their body no longer has the false stimulants such as caffeine and sugar to help 'fire' their systems throughout the day. Often what they are feeling is their *real* health and *genuine* energy levels. If this is you, don't worry; what you will find amazing is just how quickly your body starts to use its own juicy resources for energy instead of relying on short-term drug-like 'pick-me-ups'.

Although you are only on juice and smoothies, don't panic that you will collapse if you do some exercise. In fact, the opposite is true. A good walk, run, rebound, yoga session or whatever helps to clear your lymphatic system of dead cells, stimulates and focuses the mind, is a wonderful stress reliever and actually gives you more energy. What level of exercise you do is up to you, but as always use your common sense in terms of what YOU are capable and comfortable with.

Juicy Tip:
Make the 'Hot 'n' Spicy', it's delicious!

DAY 2

Juices 'n' Smoothies

7 a.m. (......)   **Hot water (with lemon, lime** or **mint)**

8 a.m. (......)   **JM's Super Juice**

11 a.m. (......)   **JM's Super Juice**

2 p.m. (......)   **JM's Super Chute Juice**

5 p.m. (......)   **JM's Turbo Express**

8 p.m. (......)   **JM's Turbo Express + 1oz wheatgrass
                   chaser** (Add a small spoonful of wheatgrass
                   powder to juice if you don't have a separate
                   wheatgrass juicer.)

9 p.m. (......)   **Fennel** or **mint tea** or **JM's Hot 'n' Spicy**

Juicy Exercise for Day 2

Morning:	1 x 20/30-minute workout
Afternoon:	1 x 15 minute-walk/run/bounce
Early Evening:	1 x 20/30-minute workout

Juicy Comments for Day 2

If you are hungry for bread, pasta and the like, remember:

It's Not **Physical** – It's **Mental!**

On a physical level, your body is getting plenty of essential good fats, amino acids (building blocks of protein), carbohydrates, vitamins, minerals, water and enzymes. If you find you are craving anything just remember it is your *mind* that is hungry at that point, not your *body*. Whatever you do, **'Don't do a Martin'** – that's my friend who had such a *mental* craving for bread that he bit a piece so hard and fast on the evening of day 2 that he actually bit a hole in his tongue! The only reason he had the craving was because he was not in the right frame of mind *first*. He attempted to do the programme with no mental preparation at all and he found it incredibly hard because of it – to the point of ending up in hospital! Don't panic. If you have followed my advice and read the book first, you will be both physically and mentally prepared, and fully aware that you are choosing to do this because YOU want to.

I have added a 15-minute workout today. If you are going to feel any 'detox' effects then this is usually the day that they hit. This is why getting as much air into your body and moving it as much as possible – as well as getting the juice/smoothies – is of paramount importance. Headaches are the most common complaint, usually caused by caffeine and refined sugar withdrawal, but it is advised you don't use any sort of drug during the programme (unless already prescribed by your GP) as you are looking to clean your system of toxins and get back some raw juicy energy!

DAY 3
Juices 'n' Smoothies

7 a.m. (......)   Hot water (with lemon, lime or mint)

8 a.m. (......)   JM's Lemon/Ginger Zinger or JM's Super Juice

11 a.m. (......) JM's Super Juice

2 p.m. (......)   Passion 4 Juice Master (*see* page 152)

5 p.m. (......)   JM's Turbo Express

8 p.m. (......)   JM's Turbo Express + 1oz wheatgrass chaser (Add a small spoonful of wheatgrass powder to juice if you don't have a separate wheatgrass juicer.)

9 p.m. (......)   Fennel or mint tea or JM's Hot 'n' Spicy

Juicy Exercise for Day 3

Morning: 1 x 30/40-minute workout
Afternoon: 1 x 20-minute walk/run/bounce
Early Evening: 1 x 30/40-minute workout

Juicy Comments for Day 3

SHOPPING DAY! You may have found that, much to your surprise, you haven't had all of the juices you could have had over the last two days. What may have surprised you even more was that this wasn't due to lack of time, but because you genuinely weren't that hungry. This comes as a real shock to most people, but if you recall I did say that most people are *overfed* but *undernourished*. Once the system starts to get raw 'live' nutrients in a liquid form it begins to be *truly* fed on a cellular level. This means that although you are consuming less you are being fed more.

In fact, you may have more provisions in your fridge than you had anticipated. If so then instead of buying all of the items on today's Shopping List (*see* page 115) you may need to adjust it accordingly. I'm also aware that some people will have had all the juices and, given the chance, would have drunk even more. Either way, tonight is shopping night, so **get prepared for the following four days in order to make sure you complete the programme.**

Juicy Tip:

If you are choosing to read the Turbo-Charge Your Life *book as part of your Phase 2 – start tonight! This will be perfect timing to have it finished by day 7 so you can start Phase 2 on day 8.*

DAY 4
Juices 'n' Smoothies

7 a.m. (......)   **Hot water (with lemon, lime or mint)**
8 a.m. (......)   JM's Super Juice
11 a.m. (......)   JM's Super Juice
2 p.m. (......)   JM's Super Detox Juice
5 p.m. (......)   JM's Turbo Express
8 p.m. (......)   **JM's Turbo Express + 1oz wheatgrass chaser** (Add a small spoonful of wheatgrass powder to juice if you don't have a separate wheatgrass juicer.)
9 p.m. (......)   **Fennel** or **mint tea** or **JM's Hot 'n' Spicy**

Juicy Exercise for Day 4

Morning: 1 x 30/40-minute workout
Afternoon: 1 x 20-minute walk/run/bounce
Early Evening: 1 x 30/40-minute workout

Juicy Comments for Day 4

Always remember, you are free to chop and change some of the juices. If you are a bit tired of a particular smoothie or juice, then have one that takes your fancy. Although they have been carefully planned to give maximum nutrients and reduce any physical withdrawal or discomfort, I have found that if your mind starts to get 'fed up' the programme can collapse. So if you do want to change one or two juices to your favourite or to one of the Extra Recipes (*see* page 181), feel free.

Juicy Tip:

If you need a little inspiration, re-read some of the testimonials, watch the DVD or listen to the 7 lbs in 7 Days motivational CD.

DAY 5
Juices 'n' Smoothies

7 a.m. (......)   **Hot water (with lemon, lime or mint)**
8 a.m. (......)   **JM's Super Chute Juice**
11 a.m. (......)   **JM's Super Chute Juice**
2 p.m. (......)   **JM's Super Detox Juice** (*see* page 144)
5 p.m. (......)   **JM's Super Juice**
8 p.m. (......)   **JM's Super Juice**
9 p.m. (......)   **Fennel or mint tea or JM's Hot 'n' Spicy**

Juicy Exercise for Day 5

Morning: 1 x 30/45-minute workout
Afternoon: 1 x 20-minute walk/run/bounce
Early Evening: 1 x 30/45-minute workout

Juicy Comments for Day 5

Most people start the programme on a Monday, so I'm
assuming today will be Friday for you. If it is, you may well
notice a 'Friday feeling' starting to creep into your head by
mid-afternoon. This is the head that says, 'Sod it, it's
Friday. Life's too short ...' and so on and so on. Personally, I
found my energy was through the roof on this day and

most people are the same. I even ran a half marathon with just one juice in my system!

The mind is your most powerful tool for success or failure. Your body is loving it – trust me, that's a given – and your mind should and can love it too. The only thing that can possibly make this difficult is if you start to bitch and moan to yourself about what you *think* you can't have. You *can* have what you want, but what you actually want is 'live' juices that will flush your system, feed your cells and help you on the journey to the land of the slim, trim and healthy – so don't ever say you can't. If in doubt ask yourself:

➤ *'How will I feel if I wake up tomorrow morning having failed?'*

Then ask:

➤ *'How will I feel when I wake up tomorrow and have succeeded yet again?'*

It's only 7 days and anyone can do anything for 7 days.

DAY 6

Juices 'n' Smoothies

7 a.m. (......)   **Hot water (with lemon, lime or mint)**
8 a.m. (......)   **Passion 4 Juice Master**
11 a.m. (......)   **Passion 4 Juice Master**
2 p.m. (......)   **JM's Pure Green Super Juice** (*see* page 156)
5 p.m. (......)   **JM's Boost Juice** (*see* page 154)
8 p.m. (......)   **JM's Boost Juice**
9 p.m. (......)   **Fennel or mint tea or JM's Hot 'n' Spicy**

Juicy Exercise for Day 6

Morning:	1 x 30/45-minute workout
Afternoon:	1 x 20-minute walk/run/bounce
Early Evening:	1 x 30/45-minute workout

Juicy Comments for Day 6

This is Saturday for most and as you can see I've changed your juicy breakfast slightly to a Passion 4 Juice Master. Trust me, this will be a most welcome change. You are almost there, but you aren't there yet. Five days is good – make no mistake – but this is a 7-day programme.

Juicy Tip:

Always be grateful for the liquid fuel you can have and not the stuff you may feel you can't. Remember, you can have whatever you like, this is YOUR choice and you are choosing to have freshly extracted juices to clean your system, test your character and change your body shape.

DAY 7
Juices 'n' Smoothies

7 a.m. (......)   **Hot water (with lemon, lime** or **mint)**

8 a.m. (......)   **JM's Super Juice**

11 a.m. (......)   **JM's Super Juice**

2 p.m. (......)   **Passion 4 Juice Master**

5 p.m. (......)   **JM's Home-made Sherbet Lemonade** (*see* page 160)

8 p.m. (......)   **JM's Boost Juice**

9 p.m. (......)   **Fennel** or **mint tea** or **JM's Hot 'n' Spicy**

Juicy Exercise for Day 7

Morning:	1 x 30/45-minute workout
Afternoon:	1 x 20-minute walk/run/bounce
Early Evening:	1 x 30/45-minute workout

Juicy Comments for Day 7

With the risk of sounding patronizing – WELL DONE! You are on the final day of juicing and tomorrow you actually get to use your teeth. What is funny is that by this stage people aren't craving junk, but their mouths are literally watering for a large salad and some rice and perhaps some fish or chicken. This is why going on to the Phase 2

Turbo Plan is so easy. Compared with a week of nothing but juices, it appears a banquet!

I sincerely hope that if you choose to weigh yourself tomorrow morning you have achieved your initial weight loss goal (BUT DON'T WEIGH YOURSELF TODAY!). I say 'initial weight loss' as I hope this is a catalyst to a life-long change for you. If you haven't done this programme to lose weight but simply to clean your system and gain more energy, again I hope you have got the result you are looking for. I look forward very much to hearing your story.

Congratulations!

You have now taken an extremely important step to Supreme Health – and a Sexy Body!

Your Juicy Journal

Throughout the week you may find it very useful to keep a diary of your progress. This will be particularly rewarding and satisfying to look back on, as well as being very useful for when you repeat '7lbs in 7 Days' in the future. We also love the juicy feedback, so please keep a few notes and let us know how you get on.

Before you start the plan it is imperative to know your weight and measurements so you will genuinely be able to evaluate your weight loss and celebrate your success. I advise you weigh yourself the first morning of the programme (usually a Monday) *before* you have a juice; and weight yourself again on the morning *after* the 7 days (day 8).

7 lbs in 7 Days Body Stats

	Day 1	Day 8
Weight		
Chest		
Waist		
Body Fat %		
Hips		

General comments about your current state of health:

I always love to hear of juicy success stories. Please e-mail your juicy stats to info@juicemaster.com

DAY 1

Today was hopefully fairly plain sailing. You should have enjoyed the novelty of just juicing and your system should feel a little emptier.

How did you find your first day of juicing?

What were the juicy highlights?

How did you get on with the juicy exercise?

How long did you do?

How did you feel?

How would you rate your overall energy level? (marks out of 10)

Any other juicy comments?

DAY 2

For some people today can be the hardest day, for others it is a breeze. Either way, having completed 48 hours you should feel great and the rest of the week should now be a piece of cake – well, not literally!

What were the juicy highlights today?

How did you get on with the juicy exercise?

How long did you do?

How did you feel?

How would you rate your overall energy level? (marks out of 10)

Any other juicy comments?

DAY 3

By now you should be feeling really juiced! Hopefully you will be starting to notice a little weight loss as well as an increase in your energy level. If you haven't noticed anything yet, then don't worry, you will – just be patient. Remember, a watched kettle never boils!

What were the juicy highlights today?

How did you get on with the juicy exercise?

How long did you do?

How did you feel?

How would you rate your overall energy level? (marks out of 10)

Any other juicy comments?

DAY 4

You are over half-way there now and you've certainly got
the finish line in your sights. More importantly, by now you
should be settled into a great rhythm and realize just how
easy and enjoyable it would be to incorporate juicing into
your daily diet long after this plan is over.

What were the juicy highlights today?

How did you get on with the juicy exercise?

How long did you do?

How did you feel?

How would you rate your overall energy level? (marks out of 10)

Any other juicy comments?

DAY 5

For many of you, today will be Friday and you might be being seduced and persuaded into indulging in fruit of the fermented variety – otherwise know as alcohol! Keep focused and remember you are *choosing* to do this: you don't *have* to do it, you *want* to do it.

What were the juicy highlights today?

How did you get on with the juicy exercise?

How long did you do?

How did you feel?

How would you rate your overall energy level? (marks out of 10)

Any other juicy comments?

DAY 6

It's the penultimate day, and you must be feeling terrific by now! Your body and mind are accustomed to your new regime and you have probably discovered there is genuinely no hunger. Many of you may only be having three or four of the juices per day, yet still feel fulfilled. This is because your body is being nourished on a cellular level above and beyond its wildest dreams – your stomach should also be feeling a lot flatter!

What were the juicy highlights today?

How did you get on with the juicy exercise?

How long did you do?

How did you feel?

How would you rate your overall energy level? (marks out of 10)

Any other juicy comments?

DAY 7

Wow, it's the last day. Just how juiced and empowered do you feel?

What were the juicy highlights today?

How did you get on with the juicy exercise?

How long did you do?

How did you feel?

How would you rate your overall energy level? (marks out of 10)

Any other juicy comments?

Your Juicy Recipes!

Juice Master's Super Juice

Juicy Ingredients
½ lime – peeled
2 Golden Delicious or Royal Gala apples
¼ pineapple
¼ medium cucumber
¼ ripe avocado
1oz of fresh wheatgrass (for other wheatgrass options, *see*
   'Wheatgrass', page 217)
1 level teaspoon of spirulina
1 capsule of acidophilus bacteria powder
Ice cubes

Juicy Instructions
Juice the apples, pineapple, cucumber and lime. Put the
avocado flesh into a blender along with the ice,
wheatgrass, spirulina, and the friendly bacteria powder.
Blend everything until smooth, pour and enjoy!

Why It's Sooooo Super!

This juice is **exploding** with some of nature's *super nutrients, enzymes, antioxidants* and *amino acids*. **Wheatgrass** and **spirulina** are two true 'super foods' which both contain a distinguished array of *vitamins* and *minerals*. The **wheatgrass** is also a rich source of chlorophyll, the undisputed top provider of *'liquid sunshine'*. It is excellent at *improving* the function of the **heart**, the **vascular system**, the **intestines** and the **lungs**, as well as *detoxifying the* **blood** and *the* **liver**. **Spirulina** is a phenomenal alga; it is supreme at harvesting the sun's energy and has been *growing naturally for more than* 3.5 **billion years!** It has been found to contain one of the most concentrated amounts of *nutrients, phytonutrients* and **antioxidants** of any plant.

This juice is exceedingly filling due to the addition of the **avocado**, which provides the body with the perfect balance of **essential fatty acids** – the *'friendly fats'* that are vital for the body!

Both the **cucumber** and the **lime** are terrific at **cleansing** the body and are **great for hair, skin and nails**.

Juice Master's Super Detox Juice

Juicy Ingredients
2 Golden Delicious or Royal Gala apples
¼ cucumber
1 stick celery
1 small handful of spinach
Ice cubes
1 heaped teaspoon of 'Power Greens' – if you don't have these,
    replace by juicing a handful of mixed green leaves
    (watercress, parsley, lettuce, etc.)

Juicy Instructions
Juice the apples, cucumber, celery and spinach. Pour into
blender, then add ice and Power Greens. Blend for about 1
minute or until smooth. If you use mixed green leaves
instead of the Power Greens, simply juice these along with
the other ingredients and the add the ice.

Why It's Sooooo Cleansing!

This is fantastic for **detoxing** and **cleansing** the system. The celery provides the body with *sodium, potassium, iron, calcium, phosphorus, magnesium, vitamin B* and *vitamin C.* Another clever property is that it **helps flush the body of excess carbon dioxide** and **reduce acidity** in the system.

Cucumber is an excellent **diuretic** and **system cleanser**; it's packed with *vitamin B, folic acid* and *calcium* and may help to *reduce cholesterol.*

This juice is *exceedingly good* for the body. Not only is it packed with *vitamins* and *minerals*, but it is also abundant in **antioxidants** and even has **anti-anaemic** and **anti-cancerous** properties.

Juice Master's Super Chute Juice™

Juicy Ingredients
2 Golden Delicious or Royal Gala apples
A small chunk of carrot
½ stick celery
1 large handful of mixed green leaves – watercress, kale, parsley,
   spinach, and whatever other green leafy veg are available
1 inch slice cucumber
½ inch of broccoli stem
1 small handful alfalfa sprouts – found in any good health shop
¼ inch slice unpeeled raw beetroot
¼ inch slice courgette (zucchini)
1 small piece of lemon – preferably, wax-free lemon with rind on
¼ inch slice ginger
2 ice cubes

Juicy Instructions
This is called a 'chute juice' because if you have a Philips
whole-fruit juicer, all you need to do is place one whole
apple in the chute followed by all the other ingredients,
finishing off with the other apple. You then simply put the
machine on the higher speed and push through. Pour over
ice. That's it and that's all! If you don't have a Philips
whole-fruit juicer, then feed all the ingredients in whatever
size the juicer will take, although clearly you may need to
cut more!

Why This Is Sooooo Special!

Not only is it fun to make this *'juice sandwich'*, but this little baby is packed with *calcium, iron, potassium, selenium, folic acid* and *chlorophyll* – the life blood of the plant – and it's like drinking *liquid sunshine!*

This juice is packed with *vitamin A*, which not only helps **maintain healthy** *skin, eyes* and *bones*, but also **boosts the** *immune system*.

Beetroot is one of nature's best *blood builders*, as well as being rich in *carotenoids*

a true anti-cancer king!

Juice Master's Turbo Express

This wonderful juice/smoothie is based on the famous Turbo-Charge Smoothie from the book *The Juice Master: Turbo-Charge Your Life in 14 Days*. This has all the nutritional elements of the TCS only in smaller amounts. This was the main juice that Katie Price (Jordan) used to lose 28 lbs in just 3 months.

Juicy Ingredients
¼ small pineapple
½ stick celery
1 inch chunk of cucumber
1 small handful spinach leaves
1 small piece of peeled lime
2 Golden Delicious or Royal Gala apples
¼ ripe avocado
Ice cubes

Juicy Instructions
Juice the pineapple, celery, cucumber, spinach, lime and apples. (If you have a Philips whole-fruit juicer, put in one apple, place other ingredients on top, and then finish up with the other apple.) Place the ripe avocado flesh in a blender/smoothie maker along with the ice and juice mixture. Give a good whiz for 45 seconds (or until smooth). Pour into glass – enjoy!

Why This Is Sooooo Turbo-Charged!

This juice is rich in *potassium, vitamin C* and *iron,* which helps **cleanse the intestine** and **boost the immune system**. It is excellent for *rebuilding red blood cells* and *reducing blood pressure*. It is also *helpful with* **kidney problems** and acts as a *diuretic*.

The blended **avocado** contains all of our body's six dietary needs in abundance – *water, fat, protein,* **natural** *sugar, vitamins* and *minerals*.

All in all, an amazing meal in a glass!

Juice Master's Hot 'n' Spicy

Juicy Ingredients
3 apples
1 good pinch of cinnamon

Juicy Instructions
Juice the apples and pour juice into a saucepan. Slowly heat but DO NOT BOIL. When nice and hot, pour into mug, add cinnamon and get cosy!

Why This Is Sooooo Hot!

This simple yet utterly delicious drink *soothes the system* and has a ***wonderfully comforting aroma***. **Apples** ooze raw life force and are considered to be one of the *finest anti-cancer and health promoters going* (growing). They are quite possibly one of the *best body cleansers* on the planet. The pectin found in the apple sweeps up and *sucks out the toxic waste* from the intestine. The humble apple also has the ability to **flush out the *liver* and *kidneys*** and help keep the *skin hydrated*.

*This warm juice is both **rewarding** to the **taste buds** and to the **tummy** – yum yum!*

Juice Master's 'Minty Beta Juice'

Don't be deceived by the simplicity of this super juice. The Beta Juice is aptly named as it's the beta-carotene king.

Juicy Ingredients
4 organic carrots
1 small handful of finely diced mint
½ level teaspoon of spirulina

Juicy Instructions
Simply juice the carrots, pour into a glass, add the mint and spirulina and stir! Yep, once again that's it and that's all!

Why This Is Sooooo Mighty Good for You!

This juice is bursting with **beta-carotene,** which is a powerful *antioxidant* and *anti-cancer queen*. It is well known that **carrots** are bursting with *beta-carotene*, but you might be surprised to know that **spirulina** has a *beta-carotene* concentration **10 times the carrot's!**
  This juice is excellent for *stimulating* and *strengthening* the **immune system** and promoting *healthy skin*. It is also terrific at *cleansing* the **liver**, helping the **digestive system**, as well as lowering **cholesterol** and *freshening the breath!*

Passion 4 Juice Master

I created this super smoothie for a juicy talk I was giving at a raw food event in the UK. A company called 'Passion4Juice' was running a juice bar there, and Trisha – owner/founder/juicette – and I made a combination smoothie which we named Passion 4 Juice Master. It is a wonderful concoction of gorgeous fruit juices, a little natural yoghurt and some super powerful nutrients supplied by a small amount of spirulina.

Juicy Ingredients
¼ small pineapple – you can juice with the skin on, but give it a
   very good wash
1 apple
¼ banana
200g natural organic yoghurt – if you're a juicy vegan, then
   simply use soya yoghurt
½ teaspoon of spirulina

Juicy Instructions
Simply juice pineapple and apple and pour into blender/smoothie maker along with the banana, yoghurt and spirulina. Blend until smooth. This will make more than an 8oz glass; drink what you want and when you are comfortably full put the rest in a flask or – as *Sesame Street* taught us – share!

Juicy Reminder:

If you don't like yoghurt (dairy or otherwise), leave it out and use ½ small pineapple instead.

Why I'm Sooooo Passionate!

This is a beautifully smooth and creamy smoothie because of the yoghurt that goes into it, and the **yoghurt** provides the body with *calcium*, which is essential for *strong bones* and *teeth*, as well as **maintaining healthy nerve function**.

The **bananas** provide an incredible source of *slow-release energy*, as well as being *rich in potassium*. This helps promote *muscle* and *nerve function* as well as *controlling blood pressure*.

Iron is one of the most common mineral deficiencies found in humans and this fantastic juice is abundant in it – thanks to the *spirulina*. It is also rich in **magnesium and trace minerals**, as well as being one of the *highest natural sources of B_{12}*.

Juice Master's Boost Juice

Juicy Ingredients
½ large pineapple
2 apples
¼ mug alfalfa sprouts
¼ mug watercress
¼ mug parsley
¼ mug kale
¼ mug broccoli
1oz shot of fresh wheatgrass juice (for other wheatgrass
    options, *see* 'Wheatgrass', page 217)
2 ice cubes

Juicy Instructions
If you have a masticating juicer, use it to juice all the
ingredients. If you have a centrifugal juicer (*see* page 207),
after juicing the apple make sure you pack the chute of
your juicer with the alfalfa, watercress, parsley, kale and
broccoli *before* turning on the machine. The tighter you
pack it and the slower you juice the more you will get out
of your centrifugal juicer. If you have a Philips whole-fruit
juicer, then all you have to do is put a whole apple in the
chute, then the kale, parsley, broccoli, alfalfa sprouts and
watercress in tight, and 'sandwich' this by putting in the
other whole apple. Then juice on the slow speed. Make
sure you allow a little time after each small push for the
juicer to work its magic. Follow by juicing the pineapple.

Add the wheatgrass shot or teaspoon of wheatgrass powder and then pour into a glass over the ice.

Note:
If adding wheatgrass powder, pour into blender with ice and blend until smooth.

Why This Is Sooooo Good!

This juice really will give you a **big boost**. It contains several natural greens including *broccoli, alfalfa sprouts, watercress, parsley* and *kale* which are some of **nature's real super-foods**. In their raw natural state these vegetables are packed with *vitamins, folic acid* and *iron*, as well as simply bursting with *chlorophyll*. This **fantastic** combination helps fight the battle against **blood pressure, liver problems** and **constipation**, as well as being a *terrific antioxidant* and *anti-cancer agent.*

Juice Master's Pure Green Super Juice

To be classed as 'pure', the ingredients for this juice in particular really should be pure and organic. This pure green juice is not for the faint-hearted on the taste front and you will need a small slice of orange in order to get your taste buds back to normal. Normally, green juices should not be drunk on their own (or only ever in small doses – as with shots of wheatgrass). However, as the two main juices are celery and cucumber, your stomach will be fine with a full glass – although I'm not sure about your taste buds! As long as you take a bite on a small slice of orange after each mouthful, all will be well. Some people's juicy taste buds have progressed to the point that they love the taste of this juice without the need for the orange, but I would play it safe for the moment.

Juicy Ingredients
2 sticks of celery
½ medium cucumber
1 small handful of spinach
1 ounce shot of fresh wheatgrass juice (or other wheatgrass
    options – *see* **'Wheatgrass', page 217)**
1 slice of orange
2 ice cubes

Juicy Instructions

Juice the celery, cucumber, spinach and wheatgrass. Add ice to a glass and pour in the super pure green juice. After each mouthful take a bite of the orange.

Juicy Tip:

Ideally all of the above should be juiced through a masticating juice extractor. If you don't have one it will still be amazing on the health and alkalizing front, but it just won't be super 'pure'. Once again, if you don't have a masticating juicer then juice the celery, cucumber and spinach and then add the wheatgrass or super green powder.

Why This Is Sooooo Pure!

Green juices **cleanse** *the system of toxins and pollutants* and can have a **rejuvenating effect** on the body. This juice is rich in *chlorophyll,* which helps to rebuild red blood cells, detoxify and purify the blood, and aid immune system function.

The **wheatgrass** contains a vast variety of *vitamins, minerals and trace elements.* Studies have shown that **1 lb of fresh** *wheatgrass* is *equal* in nutritional value to **25 lbs of fresh** *vegetables*! This juice is also wonderful for keeping your *teeth* and *gums healthy* due to the abundance of *calcium* and *vitamin C.*

Juice Master's Lemon/Ginger Zinger

This wonderful juice is a favourite of the super-fit Martina Navratilova – winner of 48 grand slam tennis tournaments. This achievement will never be rivalled and Martina is the first to put this down to her juicy ways. She has at least one freshly made juice every day, and the following is her favourite.

Juicy Ingredients
2 carrots
2 apples
1 inch slice of lemon – where possible, wax free and with the rind on
¼ inch of fresh ginger
2 ice cubes

Juicy Instructions
Simply juice the lot and pour over ice.

Why This Is Sooooo Zingerlicious!

This juice is rich in **vitamin C,** which helps *sweep up free radicals* and keeps tissues *strong* and *healthy*. The **citric acid** and **ginger** are wonderful at *eliminating toxins* from the body and *aiding digestion*. **Ginger** is also a *natural antibiotic* and one of **nature's supreme decongestants**.

This juice is full of *dietary fibre*, thanks to the simple **apple**, which oozes **vitamins and minerals**, as well as being terrific for **overall cleansing of the system**.

This juice simply *zings the* **taste buds** as well as the *liver*!

Juice Master's Home-made Sherbet Lemonade

This recipe just couldn't be easier.

Juicy Ingredients
2 Golden Delicious apples
⅓ of a lemon – where possible, wax free and with the rind on
2 ice cubes

Juicy Instructions
Simply juice the apples and lemon and pour over ice – it really does taste like sherbet lemonade!

Why This Is Sooooo Super Special

This recipe just couldn't be easier to make and the taste is *indescribable*. It's **100% natural,** with *no artificial anything* – neither you, nor your children, will never want normal sugar-loaded lemonade again!

As well as being as *easy as ABC to make*, the juice is rich in **vitamins A, B and C**, as well as *potassium, calcium, magnesium, antioxidants* and *dietary fibre*.

This lemonade is a taste sensation and is wonderful for *cleansing the system* – especially the *liver* and *kidneys*.

How to Make Natural Teas

If you can boil a kettle, then you have pretty much mastered the art of making natural teas. If you want lemon tea, simply cut a slice of lemon, place in a cup and pour on hot water. If you want mint tea, cut some fresh mint, place in a cup and pour on hot water. If you want fennel tea, cut a chunk of fresh fennel, place in a cup and pour on hot water. I think you get the picture. You can do the same for orange tea, lime tea, grape tea, peppermint tea or any kind of tea you like.

These fresh teas will play a vital role in your 7 lbs in 7 Days programme as they help to 'fire up' the stomach in the morning and help to calm the digestive tract at night.

I'll just give you one tip on this: don't fully boil the water as it can deplete the vitamin content of your drink. The rule is hot, but not boiling.

Phase 2

The Turbo-Charge Plan

The 7 lbs in 7 Days programme should have given you some amazing results in a short space of time, but if you want to make sure this 'Oh my God, my stomach feels flat' feeling remains, then it is imperative you follow the key principles of Phase 2. It is also essential that you reintroduce solid food *gradually*. Your stomach has only had liquids passing through it for a week and if you suddenly eat a three-course lunch, or binge on junk, you'll certainly know about it.

Don't Get **Stuck**

There was a show on British TV entitled *Celebrity Detox*. The programme makers took a group of 'celebrities' to Thailand for the mother of all detoxes. As reality shows go, this was a little too real to take. They showed *every* part of the celeb's detox, including them giving themselves enemas! They lived on nothing but water, fresh juices and bottom cleansing for a couple of weeks. When they arrived at the airport, the first thing one of the celebrities did was have a KFC (Kentucky Fried Chicken). As the digestive system was clean this 'food' was like a foreign invader and it 'blocked' him up. Apparently, he couldn't go to the toilet for a week and was in great pain. His body simply wasn't ready to go from pure natural juices to KFC – it needed time to adjust (although I don't think I could ever adjust to KFC!).

This demonstrates that it is essential that even if you think you want to do whatever you think would be cool for you on the food front during Phase 2, make sure that for the first couple of days you ease in gently by having light foods such as fruit, steamed vegetables, salads, soups, rice, tofu, yoghurt and so on. This will help to increase your metabolic rate *slowly* to meet the new demand. If you are patient it will soon reach the stage where it is ready for and can easily handle cooked food again.

PURE REACTIONS

You have been having nothing but 'raw' food and so your body is probably purer than it's been in years. The purer your system is, the more sensitive it becomes to anything which may endanger its overall health. For example, if you were to give a non-smoker a cigarette and ask them to inhale it, they would either cough, splutter, retch or actually be sick. But give a cigarette to someone who already smokes and ask them to inhale and they – on the surface, anyway – will have no adverse physical reactions. In fact, often if a smoker is coughing slightly and they take a few drags of a cigarette they *stop* coughing! Why? Because when the body detects a poison – as in the case of tobacco – it will have an *immediate* reaction to inform the person that what they are doing is harmful to the system. If, however, the person overrides the signals and continues to smoke, the body will learn that for whatever reason it has no choice and will adjust accordingly.

The human body is one of the most efficient survival machines on Earth and, despite what you throw at it, it will do anything within its power to make sure you stay alive. Survival comes first – health second. It soon stops giving health warning signals to the smoker and does whatever it can to make the process feel as comfortable as possible while at the same time doing what it can to filter out the 4,000 poisonous chemicals contained in the average cigarette. If someone stops smoking for a long period of time and then suddenly inhales one, they will get almost the same adverse physical reactions as when they first started.

The same principle applies with food. If your system is 'clean' you will be much more sensitive to processed food and to large amounts of food. Your system will also need to work harder to digest, assimilate and dispose of the waste from processed food than it does from nature's finest – especially when nature's finest has been juiced and blended. So ...

LET YOUR METABOLIC RATE INCREASE
NATURALLY

This is one of the main reasons people put on so much weight so quickly after they stop any kind of detox plan. They are often 'hanging on in there' in a diet mentality so when the detox plan is over – BOOM – they immediately think they are a success and try to eat the entire contents of a supermarket in one sitting. The system just isn't ready for it, the metabolism isn't ready for it. Because the metabolism has been used to pre-digested food –

pre-digested by the plant and then juiced or blended – it has had very little work to do and so the metabolism has *decreased* according to demand. This is why if it goes straight from freshly extracted juices to something like a large meal of KFC, or a big bowl of cereal with several rounds of toast followed by a cooked breakfast, it will struggle and weight will be put on again ... *fast!*

This is why I strongly recommend that if you do decide to skip the whole of the Phase 2 Turbo-Charge Plan, you make sure you eat easy-to-digest foods to fire up your metabolism again. It will take a couple of days for your system to build up its 'metabolic muscles', so reintroduce solid food slowly. However, the following Phase 2 Turbo-Charge Plan is the perfect way for your system to readjust.

On with the Plan

I have entitled Phase 2 the 'Turbo-Charge Plan' as it is based on my previous book *The Juice Master: Turbo-Charge Your Life in 14 Days*. I advised you to read this book during the 7lbs in 7 Days programme. In fact, the book was on your midweek shopping list. I am pleased to say that most people do get round to reading the book and in doing so find that not only do they have a comprehensive day-by-day, recipe-by-recipe plan of exactly what to do for the next two weeks and beyond – they also get re-inspired. I don't just mean re-inspired to eat well, but the book acts as a catalyst to other major life changes.

The combined results of people doing the 7 lbs in 7 Days followed by *Turbo-Charge Your Life in 14 Days* has been breathtaking. Here's one letter as a single example:

> 'Thank you, thank you, thank you! I took your advice and read the Turbo book while on 7-day juice diet. I did both programmes and have lost 18 lbs! I also feel alive again and I have a new-found respect for myself and my life ... I cannot thank you enough.'

If you didn't read the Turbo-Charge book, either grab yourself a copy (library, borrow from a friend, buy, beg, etc.) or follow the Turbo-Charge principles.

The Turbo-Charge Principles

Days 8–10

Breakfast: Veggie-based juice/smoothie breakfast (your choice).

Lunch: Veggie-based juice/smoothie, or good avocado salad, or fruit salad.

Dinner: Large salad, or wholegrain/wild rice with steamed vegetables, or fish with salad or veggies, or 'lite bite' rye toast with avocado sardine (or tuna), or your own recipe based on these principles.

Days 11–21

Breakfast: Juice/smoothie, or fruit, or porridge oats with fruit; or rye toast with Manuka honey, or 'live' yoghurt.

Lunch: Juice/smoothie, or fruit, or big pot of 'live' yoghurt, or 2 slices of rye toast with avocado or fish, or stuffed wholemeal pitta bread with salad and whatever takes your fancy, or large avocado, feta cheese or whatever salad you like.

Dinner: Large salad, or wholegrain/wild rice with steamed vegetables, or fish with salad or veggies, or 'lite bite' rye toast with avocado sardine (or tuna), or freshly made soup, or your own recipe based on these principles.

Key Turbo Principles

The above guidelines are just that – guidelines. After you follow days 8–10 to the letter, you can be slightly more flexible with days 11–21 as long as you keep to the following key principles.

Exercise

For those who have read the Turbo-Charge book you will
know that exercise features prominently. You may or may
not have been doing some exercise during the 7 lbs
programme, but whether you have or not, this is the time
to step it up a little.

Here's the exercise plan for Phase 2:

Morning:	30/45 mins
Evening:	30/45 mins

That's it! What you do is up to you, but the body was
designed to MOVE. Remember, the quickest and easiest
way to feel alive in the morning or after work is to move.
Let's not forget that not moving at all means you are dead!
Life breeds life and exercise is the quickest and easiest way
to relieve tension and clean the system. So hop, skip, jump,
run, yoga, bounce or whatever – just move!

Breakfast

I have suggested a juice or smoothie during this time, but
feel free to be flexible. Oats, rye toast, the odd egg, 'live'
yoghurt are all OK. If you can keep to the juices for
breakfast, though, so much the better.

Lunch

If you are going to choose things such as stuffed wholemeal pittas, then lunch is the time to have them. I suggest that during Phase 2 any man-made carbs (with the exception of rice) are eaten during the day. These would include wholegrain bread, wholegrain pasta, sweet potatoes and the like. There are many options for lunch, such as rice, yoghurt, rye bread, pitta bread, salad and soup, but many people simply keep to something like a Super Juice for breakfast, a Turbo Smoothie for lunch and a nice protein-rich dinner. This was exactly the system that Katie Price (Jordan) followed when she dropped 28 lbs in three months.

Dinner

The evening meal is protein rich combined with high-water-content natural food. In other words, something like hot fish on a large bed of avocado salad or some organic chicken with steamed veggies. The only carb, other than vegetables, that I recommend during Phase 2 is wholegrain/wild rice. One of the best meals on the planet on a nutritional front is rice and veggies. In fact, the countries where the people live the longest tend to have a diet rich in rice and vegetables.

The key is imagination and flexibility. This book is a 7-day juice programme, but I couldn't not give some guidelines on what to do afterwards. I realize I haven't given a complete recipe guide for Phase 2, but this is where you need to use your imagination or go to a library and look at the recipes in *The Juice Master: Turbo-Charge Your Life in 14 Days*. Alternatively, I have put some on the website: **www.juicemaster.com**

Some people choose to carry on eating this way until they have reached their optimum health and weight, others want a little more flexibility. With that in mind let's move on to Phase 3 ...

Phase 3
The Juicy Lifestyle

Be F*L*EX*I*B*L*E and Let Common Sense Prevail

I am sure that most people are under the impression that
nothing other than juice ever passes my lips. I can assure
you that this is *far* from the case, as those who know me
well will testify. I *love* eating all kinds of things, and I love
tasting what many different countries and cultures have to
offer. I used to be quite obsessed by food and I was also
quite a strict vegan. I personally found this 'label' fairly
restricting as it often prevented me from indulging in the
many delights life has to offer. I now have total freedom
around all food and use juicing as a tool, a catalyst if you
will, to ensure that I keep the weight off and a good flow of
nutrients in. I do the 7lbs in 7 days Juice Cleanse at least
once every three months and have a nothing-but-juice day
once a week. I eat only when I am genuinely hungry, stop
eating when I'm full and make sure that very little 'junk'
enters my system. I also exercise every day in order to keep
mobile and avoid 'seizing up'. In addition, exercise keeps
my metabolism high, cleanses my lymphatic system, and
helps to keep me lean and feeling good.

However, I also make sure that I am totally free to try
any food and not be rude to a host who has spent time and
money making a dish for me. Freedom around food is the
key to Phase 3 and permanent weight loss. It's also the key
to retaining your sanity! No matter how good the 7 days
have made you feel, my intention is not to turn you into a
'juicearian' or a 'juicearexic' (if there are indeed such

things). We have teeth for a reason and good-quality food is essential for optimum health. The 7-day plan is a simple clean-out, not a way of life. Phase 2 is the necessary follow-up to it, and Phase 3 is all about being flexible and doing what is needed for lifelong success.

It's Not **All** About the Juice

If you have completed the 7lbs in 7 days and the Turbo-Charge programmes (and if you haven't, please stop reading this and return to it once you have!), there is no way on Earth you won't be feeling a damn sight better than you did three weeks ago. Having witnessed thousands of people go through these programmes, it's safe to say you will be feeling on fire. The last thing you'll wish is for that fire to go out, so it's now time to continue with your juicy lifestyle and make sure you don't go back to your old ways. A juicy lifestyle is not one where you are obsessed with food or image. A juicy lifestyle is one where you feel mentally and physically juiced on a *daily* basis; where you *want* to do things, as opposed to feeling that you *have* to do them. It's a lifestyle where you feel slim, trim and light while not being obsessed with food. As long as you keep to the 'Key Juicy Lifestyle Principles', which I will be laying out in a sec, you'll be flying for life.

I personally lost my excess weight and turned my health around over a decade ago. I am *not* always 100 per cent 'good' and, because of this, I get to taste all of what life has to offer. However, I *am* an advocate of the Key Principles and they keep me in shape, both mentally and physically. If you do slip up on massive scale for whatever reason and feel yourself expanding in the wrong way, it's comforting to know you are only ever 7 days away from a major change and dramatic weight loss. I know many people who do the 7 days twice or four times a year, and many do as I do and have a 'juice day' once a week.

> *I've been fat and I've been slim –*
> *Trust me, slim wins ...* **every time!**

Please do not underestimate the effect that being able to wear whatever you want, whenever you want, will have on your confidence. And do not underestimate the effect that feeling light and being able to move will have on your life. I sincerely hope you keep this juicy feeling, adopt it as a lifestyle, and achieve your weight and health goals, if you haven't done so already. I love hearing of people's successes, so if you feel like sharing yours please write to me at info@juicemaster.com. Alternatively, perhaps I'll see you at a retreat one day and you can share your story with me personally. Until then ... stay juiced!

Key Juicy Lifestyle Principles

➤ 60–80% of what you consume should consist of high-water-content 'live' foods – fruits, vegetables, juices and smoothies – with the remainder being made up of lean proteins (fish and chicken), wholegrain carbs (rice, bread, potatoes), nuts, seeds, and some dairy products if you so wish.

➤ Eat your food *slowly*.

➤ Drink your juices and smoothies *slowly*.

➤ Never eat if you aren't *genuinely* hungry – no matter what the clock says!

➤ Exercise once or twice a day with a combined time of *at least* 45 mins.

➤ Do the 7-day programme once every season.

➤ Feel grateful for all the benefits you enjoy.

➤ Watch no more than 1 hour of TV a day.

➤ Watch an inspirational film or documentary once a week.

➤ Read a book every two weeks.

➤ Do something thoughtful for someone else every day.

➤ Be flexible around food and *never* label yourself – vegan/vegetarian/etc.

➤ Don't forget to go and PLAY!

To make your Juicy Lifestyle even more enjoyable, I've added some more recipes for you to try out. Have fun!

Juicy Recipes for Life

Juice Master's Fruity Zest

Juicy Ingredients
¼ pineapple
½ inch slice lemon – unwaxed, with the rind on
3 strawberries
1 small handful raspberries
½ banana

Juicy Instructions
Juice the pineapple and lemon. Place the strawberries, raspberries and banana into the blender, add the juice and blend until smooth.

Juice Master's Morning Magic

Juicy Ingredients
½ stick celery
1 inch cucumber
2 apples
¼ lime
¼ avocado
½ teaspoon spirulina
2 ice cubes

Juicy Instructions
Juice the celery, cucumber, apples and lime. Place the flesh of the avocado, the spirulina and ice into the blender, add the juice and blend until smooth.

Juice Master's Rehydration Crush

Juicy Ingredients
2 mugs diced watermelon
4 crushed ice cubes

Juicy Instructions
Simply place ingredients into blender and blend until smooth.

Juice Master's Simply Canteloupe

Juicy Ingredients
⅓ medium canteloupe melon
1 small handful crushed ice

Juicy Instructions
Wash but DO NOT PEEL the melon. Juice with the skin on and pour over ice. Sounds simple but the taste is divine!

Juice Master's Simply Red

Juicy Ingredients
¼ pineapple
1 apple
¼ inch slice lemon
½ inch slice courgette
1 inch slice red pepper
1 inch chunk *raw* beetroot
2 ice cubes

Juicy Instructions
Juice all the ingredients and pour over ice.

Juice Master's Muesli Smoothie

Juicy Ingredients
¼ pineapple
2 apples
3 strawberries
½ banana
2 tablespoons 'live' natural yoghurt – if vegan, replace with
   soya yoghurt
1 small handful organic muesli
3 ice cubes

Juicy Instructions
Juice the pineapple and apple. Place the strawberries,
banana, natural yoghurt, ice and muesli into the blender,
add the juice and blend until smooth.

Juice Master's 3-Seed Smoothie

Juicy Ingredients

3 tablespoons 'live' yoghurt – if vegan, replace with soya
    yoghurt
1 tablespoon 3-seed mix – obtain natural sunflower, pumpkin
    and sesame seeds from health shop or supermarket, and mix
    in equal proportions
2 large oranges – peeled, but keep the white 'pith' on
½ peeled banana
1 teaspoon honey – Manuka or other 'active' honey
Pinch of cinnamon
6 ice cubes

Juicy Instructions

Juice the oranges. Pour orange juice into blender with all
other ingredients and blend until smooth.

Juice Master's Vanilla, Honey and Live Yoghurt Smoothie

This tastes soooooooooooooooooooooooooooooo good!

Juicy Ingredients
½ teaspoon honey – Manuka or similar 'active' honey
½ teaspoon vanilla essence
300g of 'live' yoghurt – if vegan, replace with soya yoghurt
4 ice cubes

Juicy Instructions
Simply place all ingredients in blender, and whiz until smooth.

Juice Master's Totally Tropical Taste

This gorgeous juice is a completely natural version of a popular soft drink. The ingredients are simple but the taste and texture are divine.

Juicy Ingredients
½ small pineapple
1 ruby grapefruit – peeled, but leave the pith on
4oz of sparkling spring water
Ice

Juicy Instructions
Juice the pineapple and grapefruit, add the water and pour over ice.

Juice Master's Super Workout & Recovery Juice

The late Dr Norman Walker, one of the world's leading juice pioneers, was a great believer in this juice. He believed the combination was the perfect balance of sodium and potassium – two vital minerals that we lose while working out. The Super Workout Juice should be taken around 30 minutes before a workout and then at some point during the first hour afterwards. This juice helps with the aches and pains usually associated with exercise.

Juicy Ingredients
¼ small cucumber
1 stick celery
2 apples
Ice

Juicy Instructions
Juice the lot and pour over ice.

Juicy Tip:
Make and put in flask and take to gym.
After your workout, drink while relaxing in the sauna!

Juice Master's Iced Mango Crush

Juicy Ingredients
1 large ripe mango
½ peeled pineapple
1 lime
1 cup of crushed ice

Juicy Instructions
De-stone and peel mango. Cut lime in half. Juice the
pineapple. Add juice, mango flesh and crushed ice to
blender. Squeeze lime juice over all and blend until
smoothie.

Juice Master's Athlete's Elixir

The best forms of carbohydrates on the planet are fruits and vegetables. Many athletes feel they need loads of pasta and bread before a major event, but having completed a triathlon myself with only the following juice inside me, I know first hand that nature knows best. I would suggest having this an hour before an event and then again afterwards.

Juicy Ingredients
2 apples
1 stick of celery
1 banana
3 pitted dates
½ teaspoon honey – Manuka or similar 'active' honey
Ice

Juicy Ingredients
Juice apples and celery and pour into blender with all other ingredients. Whiz until smooth.

Juice Master's Protein Power-House Smoothie

Calling all weight-lifters and thin people – here's a protein power smoothie designed to fill you out in all the right places.

Juicy Ingredients
4 almonds
4 brazil nuts
2 pitted dates
2 bananas
1 small handful sesame seeds
1 handful blueberries – frozen or fresh
300g 'live' natural yoghurt – if vegan, replace with soya yoghurt
¼ teaspoon vanilla essence
8 ice cubes

Juicy Instructions
Simply put the whole lot in the blender and whiz until thick and smooth. This really is a meal in a glass.

Juice Master's '5 Portions in a Glass' Smoothie

We hear all the time that we must have 5 portions of fruits and veg a day, but how many of us actually get around to having them? I call this delicious smoothie '5 portions in a glass', but as the official guidelines stand, no matter how many different combinations of fruit and veg you have, if it's in the form of a juice it only ever counts as one portion. This clearly is nonsense but, hey, the law is the law. Anyway, if you have just one glass each day you will be getting more genuine nutrition than most people get in a month.

Juicy Ingredients
2 apples
¼ pineapple
1 inch slice courgette
½ avocado
1 stick celery
1 inch slice cucumber – diced
1 lime

Juicy Instructions
Juice 1½ of the apples along with the pineapple, celery and courgette. Dice the rest of the apple and place into blender along with diced cucumber and ice. Blend until thick and smooth.

Juicy Tip:
If this is too thick for you, add a little
mineral water and blend again.

Juice Master's Kids' Veggie Special

Can't get your kids to eat their veg? Well, ever thought about getting them to drink them? This is a way of mixing some highly nutritious vegetable juices with fruit so that the kids never know they are drinking live vegetable juice. Just don't tell them what's really in it!

Juicy Ingredients
1 small *raw* beetroot
2 Apple – Golden Delicious or similar
¼ small pineapple
1 stick celery
1 small handful spinach
1 inch slice cucumber
Ice

Juicy Instructions
Simply juice the lot and pour over ice! The beetroot will make this juice very red so you can tell the kids it's some kind of berry juice – sometimes a little white lie can be for the good.

Juice Master's Salad Juice

If the thought of eating salads is a bit much, ever thought of drinking them? Sounds a bit odd but don't knock it till you've tried!

Juicy Ingredients
1 large handful rocket, watercress and spinach leaves
1 small tomato
1 inch slice cucumber
3 medium carrots
1 inch piece fresh ginger
Ice

Juicy Instructions
Juice everything and pour over ice.

Juicy Tip:
Make sure you pack the salad leaves into the chute of the juicer and then turn it on and push through slowly. If juicing with a masticating juicer, just juice with the machine on.

Juice Master's Chunky Funky Monkey

A chocolate feel, with a banana and vanilla taste – gorgeous!

Juicy Ingredients
1 banana
¼ spoon vanilla essence
1 teaspoon carob powder
250g 'live' yoghurt – if vegan, replace with soya yoghurt
6 almonds
1 teaspoon honey – Manuka or other 'active' honey
4 ice cubes

Juicy Instructions
Place everything in blender and whiz until smooth.

Juice Master's Summer Smoothie

Juicy Ingredients
8 fresh strawberries
2 oranges – peeled but keep the pith on
¼ lemon
4 ice cubes

Juicy Instructions
Juice the oranges and lemon. Place the strawberries and ice into blender and pour in the juice. Blend until smooth.

Cool as a Cucumber

Cucumber is nature's natural cooler and the juice is perfect for those hot summer days.

Juicy Ingredients
½ small cucumber
1 stick celery
¼ medium pineapple
2 ice cubes

Juicy Instructions
Juice the lot and pour over ice.

More **Juicy** Help

The Power of a Coach

During the 7 days, there won't be too many people who are supporting you. In fact, such is the way of the world, if someone sees somebody else trying to improve their lives, instead of supporting them, they have a tendency to drag them down.

This isn't usually done out of malice and isn't even a conscious reaction but, nonetheless, it does happen and you need to be aware of it. The reality is that if someone thinks it's too difficult to improve their own house, they will want to try and knock yours down, especially if you're making massive improvements. After all, the better your house looks the more aware they become of the state theirs is in.

This is why I've devised the *7 lbs in 7 Days* CD, DVD and app. The app has audio and video coaching, the shopping list, and all the videos of how to make the juices and smoothies. It may sound like a piece of cake going on juices

only for 7 days (or maybe not!), but trust me, there will be
a few 'Sod it' moments on the programme and this is
where you need to be able to tap into the right psychology
in that particular moment. When running the 7lbs in 7
Days Super Juice Detox Retreats, usually miles away from
anywhere – up a mountain, near the sea – I'm aware of
how much easier it is. For one thing, I, or a member of the
team, is on hand to help coach you throughout the week,
and for another, even if you did want to run off and get a
burger and fries it's almost impossible for you to do so
(unless you're into mountain climbing or can swim 30
miles in the sea!). The CD/DVD and/or app aren't
essential, but if you want to make this process even easier,
then it's worth having your own virtual 'Juice Coach' for a
week. That way you won't feel like you're doing it alone
and, as most people do this once a season, you always
have the CD/DVD or app for future occasions.

'Oh, I'll Come on It **with** You'

Now you may think that if you go on the programme with
someone, then you won't be on your own either, but one
thing is for sure – when it comes to this sort of thing

You Are Always Pretty Much on Your **Own**

Unless you are with them 24/7, you have no idea if they are
actually doing the programme to the letter (or they you),
and very often the strength in numbers philosophy rarely

applies with a programme of this nature. The reality is that if you decide to do the programme with a friend (as you well might) it can go one of two ways. You both either fully support each other, find the process easy, and look and feel amazing in a week. Or one of you starts cracking and in your panic starts to do some negative coaching, usually along the lines of, *'This is stupid. Come on, you've got to eat, there's no way this is normal – or healthy!'* In other words, they will do anything to try to rope you into their negative way of thinking in order to justify having a quick binge and writing off the whole programme. You may even find that it's not them doing it – but you!

This is why I would advise that if you are going to do this with someone, please never be influenced by their negative thinking or their justifications. If they want to give in, then that's cool, but you are doing this programme for you; for *your* health, *your* weight, *your* energy, and *your* life. What they choose to do is their call, just don't get roped into it the usual spiral of negative chit-chat.

Your 10 Steps to Quick and Easy Juicing

1 Place all the ingredients you need for your recipe on your chopping board before you do anything else.

2 Place a biodegradable pulp bag in the 'pulp container' of your juicer. (If you don't have any Juice Master biodegradable pulp bags, just use a carrier bag.) This will help as this will be one less part to clean. *Note:* Not all juicers have separate pulp containers.

3 Prepare, wash and, if you need to (depending on your juicer), cut the produce into pieces small enough to go into the chute of your juicer. Put back into the fridge any produce not required for the recipe. If you have any ingredients which need blending as part of the recipe, add them to your blender at this stage.

4 Half fill the sink with warm soapy water.

5 Turn on the juice extractor and juice everything in one go.

6 Put the jug of juice to one side *before* cleaning. (If you are making a smoothie, then pour the juice into the

blender and blend until smooth, then pour and leave the glass to one side.) Make it a rule not to drink your juice until you have cleaned the machine.

7 Undo the machine, scoop out the pulp from the lid of the machine and place it into the bag that's in the pulp container (or into the rubbish bin if you don't have a separate pulp container on your juicer). Throw the bag into the bin or, preferably, put it aside for composting.

8 Put all the parts of the machine (except the electrical unit) into the sink.

9 Most parts of the machine will simply rinse clean with warm running water. The mesh/filter part will need attention with a washing brush (or nail brush) in order to clean it effectively. It is very important that this part is cleaned properly in order to extract the maximum juice from future uses.

10 Quickly run a tea towel over the machine, put it back together and return everything to your 'Juice Station', where it's once again inviting to use.

How to Set Up Your Home Juice Bar

Having your very own juice and smoothie bar at home is perhaps the best thing you can do for yourself and your family's health. Not only does it look funky, but you are much more likely to get some very good quality 'raw', 'live' nutrition into your system on a daily basis if you have your own juice bar – ready to use – in your house. When it comes to this programme, I would say it's essential. If you have a copy of my *Funky Fresh Juice Book*, it has a cool illustration in colour of exactly how your funky juice bar should look. If you don't, I'll do my best to put it across in black-and-white words here.

Juicing Is for Life – so Make It Easy!

The key to having a successful juice bar at home is organizing your space. With more and more kitchen gadgets coming onto the market, worktop space is becoming increasingly scarce. The mistake that most people make when they start juicing is that because they feel other kitchen gadgets should take priority, they tend to put the juicer in the cupboard after its first use. The problem with this is that:

➤ You are much more likely to forget the juicer is there.
➤ If you do want to juice you have to clear space every time – meaning you probably won't bother.
➤ Juicing will never become routine.

I have yet to enter a kitchen, no matter how small, that couldn't fit in a home juice and smoothie station. All it requires is a little imagination and letting go of some clutter. You will be amazed at just how little we use many of the items on our work surface. Just as most of us only wear 20% of our clothes 80% of the time, it's similar with the bits and pieces on the worktop.

If you are anything like the people who have done this programme before, the chances are you will be juicing for much longer than the 7 days. Most people continue to some degree throughout their life. With this in mind, it's clearly worth getting your home juice bar right at the outset.

The first thing you need to do is to take a good look at your kitchen and remove what you really don't need. Remember that bread maker you bought at the good food show last year? Get rid of it. You certainly won't be needing that deep-fat fryer again. And if you have a microwave that sits on the worktop, why not find somewhere for it out of the way while you are doing the 7-day plan. If your children have their food heated and cooked in it, then you'll be doing them a favour if you get rid of it for a while at least. Fresh is always best, so while you are feeding yourself super nutrients, give the kids some fresh food too.

Setting Up Your Juice Bar Couldn't Be Easier

➤ **Your juicer and blender/smoothie maker** should take pride of place. They need to be in an easy-to-use position. If you do need to put them to the back of the work surface, then make sure they are easy to pull forward for easy use. Make sure that your juicer and blender are together – don't put one at one side of your kitchen and the other at the other end. Make it easy for yourself.

➤ **Your chopping board** wants to be next to where you have your juicer and blender. This is important for speed of juicing and convenience.

➤ **Always have a good sharp knife** ready to use on the chopping board or very near the juice bar. Have a **clean tea towel** on the chopping board or near it.

➤ Make sure you have plenty of room and NO CLUTTER around your juice bar.

➤ Pin up the **7 lbs in 7 Days wall planner** near your juice bar for easy recipe reference.

➤ And finally – ALWAYS KEEP THE AREA CLEAN AND READY FOR USE.

Which Juicer?

Getting the right juicer is crucial to your success on this programme *and* beyond. For our purposes, there are just two basic types of juicer:

➤ Masticating
➤ Centrifugal

The most common by far is the **centrifugal** type. In fact, at the time of writing this book you cannot buy a masticating juicer in the high street, so the chances are that you will only have seen centrifugal juicers. I will cover masticating juices in a bit, but as centrifugal juicers are by far the most common – and probably the one you'll get – I have mainly concentrated on this group.

A centrifugal juicer has a fast-rotating cutting blade. This blade chops the fruit and veg into pieces before throwing them forcefully against a filter that in turn separates the juice from the fibre. This type of juicer is more than adequate for this programme and everyday juicing. Many choose to get a centrifugal juicer and a separate wheatgrass juicer, which I'll also explain in a second. But first, what centrifugal juicer should you get?

There are many centrifugal juicers on the market today, but they aren't all built the same. Choosing which centrifugal juicer to buy has always been tricky, and it often came down to budget and how many people you were juicing for. I would say that even if you own a juicer, you just may want to treat yourself to an upgrade. In my view, the choice has now become a one-horse race.

Philips – Sense and Simplicity

Whoever was in charge of making Philips's top-end range of juicers knew exactly what they were doing. They not only look about as slick as it gets – and yes they do look good – but they have a wide chute. Now if you've never juiced this may not seem like a big deal, but you can put up to three WHOLE apples in without *any* chopping, coring or peeling! In fact it was after using the Philips Alu for the first time that I created my now famous Chute Juice, which is featured in the 7 lbs in 7 Days programme. It's the one where you simply fill the chute with whatever fruit and veg take your fancy, turn on the machine, push through and boom – a full glass of juice in one easy hit.

But the wide chute and slick aesthetics are not what makes this juicer stand head and shoulders above the rest. We all want a juicer that extracts as much juice as possible from the fruit and vegetables – this has always been a big problem with wide-chute juicers. Although they could take a whole apple with no chopping, coring or peeling, the motors were often not up to the job and many simply blew out during the first few months of use. And on top of this, they were just rubbish at extraction. Many people were willing to put up with less extraction for the speed and convenience of a wide-chute juicer. However, this is no longer necessary.

Philips have a new patented extraction mechanism which has been shown to extract as much as 70% more juice than some conventional juicers, which constitutes a considerable saving in terms of time and money. The 70% test must have been against some very small machines, but even when up against all the other latest wide-chute juicers the Philips produces MUCH more juice. The Juice Master Team conducted its own survey using a range of juicer models and in our tests the Philips Alu juicer produced 20% *more* juice than any other juicer on the market.

Philips are clearly not the only company that make juicers, but at the time of writing their juicers are the best. This is also the opinion of *Which?* magazine and *Good Housekeeping*. If you are reading this outside the UK, look out for the Juice Master's Funky Fresh Juicer Collection, which should be out very soon in some very funky colours! However, as I do not know when and where you will be reading this, please always make a point of looking at my site for what's hot in the juice-extractor world *before* you buy your machine.

Masticating and Wheatgrass Juicers

A masticating juicer is a completely different animal from the centrifugal type. The quality of the juice they produce tends to be a lot better due to the way they extract it, but better quality comes at a price.

With regard to the financial cost, the best twin-gear masticating juicers cost anywhere from £250 to £450. Personally, I think the extra cost is more than justified as not only is the quality and extraction of the juice better, but because they extract the juice *slowly* the oxidation is much slower. This means that the high nutritional quality of the juice lasts much longer, so you can make juice the night before for the following day. However, as well as the financial implications there are also time implications. Compared to a centrifugal juicer, masticating juicers, especially the Philips whole-fruit model, can take a great deal of time to make a juice.

It's worth knowing that, with the exception of the 'Champion' juicer, **all masticating juicers also juice**

wheatgrass. A good masticating juicer will also extract the most from green leafy veg and herbs such as alfalfa, parsley, mint, kale, broccoli, spinach, watercress and so on. Many people who do this programme use the Philips whole-fruit juicer together with a separate manual or electric wheatgrass juicer.

The choice of what juicer to get really does come down to budget and time. There are many masticating juicers on the market today, but like centrifugal juicers, they're not all built the same. Before buying any juicer please feel free to call the juicy team for advice (0845 130 28 29) or visit **www.juicemaster.com.**

Which Blender/ Smoothie Maker?

A blender and a smoothie maker are one and the same thing. It was Kenwood who managed to get people who already owned a blender to go out and also buy a smoothie maker. So many people think they are somehow different, but in realty it is like calling a pan an 'egg boiler'!

There are many good blenders on the market these days but there are also some terrible models out there. When buying a blender you want to make sure it can blend ice and *frozen* fruits with speed and ease. One thing you don't want for this programme is a hand-blender – you need one with a plastic or glass jug.

To see my full recommendations, go to **www.juicemaster.com** or call the juicy team (0845 130 28 29).

Super Foods

Spirulina

What is spirulina?

Even my computer's spell-check doesn't recognize it. It is in fact an alga that's been growing on this Earth for over 3.5 billion years. Interesting, but why would you want to consume such an ancient and unappealing plant and what possible benefit could this have on your health? Believe it or not, spirulina is actually ...

*One of the Healthiest **Super** Foods to be Found on the **Planet!***

The foods we eat defend our body from the negative effects of lifestyle stress, pollution, radiation and toxic chemicals.

Yet many processed foods are nutritionally empty and therefore leave us vulnerable to poor health and low energy levels. The good news is that many essential nutrients recommended by experts to help protect our bodies can be found in high concentrations in spirulina. In fact, it contains the most powerful combination of nutrients known in any grain, herb or food, so this really is one of nature's superheroes on the nutrition front.

This tiny aquatic plant is simply amazing: it consists of 60% protein, it is bursting with essential vitamins and phytonutrients, such as the antioxidant beta-carotene and the rare essential fatty acid GLA, as well as containing numerous other essential nutrients. Its deep-green colour comes from its rainbow of natural pigments – chlorophyll (green), phycocyanin (blue) and carotenoids (orange). All in all, this little aquatic magician can quite literally harvest the sun's energy, so that you and I can virtually be drinking liquid sunshine! Spirulina is:

➤ **The world's highest beta-carotene food** – Carrots are famous for their nutritional value, principally due to their high beta-carotene content, but it might surprise you to know that spirulina has a beta-carotene concentration of 10 TIMES THAT OF THE CARROT, its nearest rival.

➤ **60% easy-to-digest vegetable protein without any fat or cholesterol** – We are increasingly aware of the importance of lowering the amount of cholesterol and fat in our diets. In order to do this many people are consuming far less meat and dairy protein. Spirulina is the highest natural protein food containing all the essential amino acids that the body requires, but with none of the cholesterol or saturated fats associated with meat and dairy products.

➤ **One of only two whole foods that contain a rare essential fatty acid** – Gamma-linolenic acid (GLA) is a rare essential fatty acid found in the Omega-6 family. It is present in mother's milk which helps with the development of healthy babies, and it continues to have a wide range of health-promoting properties throughout our life. Studies show nutritional deficiencies can block GLA production in the body, so a good dietary source of GLA can be important. Spirulina is the only other whole food that contains GLA.

➤ **Abundant in iron** – Iron deficiency is the most common mineral deficiency, yet it is essential for the body to build a strong system. 40% of women under 50 are deficient in iron. Spirulina is not only rich in iron but it is also contained in a form much easier to absorb than the iron found in supplements.

➤ **Bursting with vitamin B-12 and B complex** – Spirulina is the richest source of B-12, essential for healthy nerves and tissues; this is especially important for vegetarians.

Health Warning: Spirulina Can Seriously Benefit Your Health

This super food of the 1990s is not a synthetic laboratory concoction, but is naturally occurring and has been used throughout history to nourish people in Africa and America. Today, spirulina is consumed on a regular basis by health-conscious people all over the world and is probably the most extensively researched food micro-alga. Many people incorporate spirulina into their regular diet due to its amazing health advantages, which besides nutritional health insurance include increased energy, internal cleansing, as well as helping with weight control. Spirulina can be used to supplement the power of the foods you eat, but you can also lean on it when you can't eat, or when you don't eat the foods you know you should in order to boost your bodies natural defences. The experience of long-term consumers and the scientific evidence suggest that taking spirulina on a daily basis will provide significant health benefits. Therefore mixing a teaspoon of spirulina into your daily juice or smoothie is possibly one of the easiest and simplest forms of health insurance you can buy into. (*See* **www.juicemaster.com** for more details.)

Wheatgrass

'1 lb of fresh wheatgrass is equal in nutritional value to nearly 25 lbs of other green vegetables.'

Anne Wigmore

Drinking grass is not everyone's cup of tea! I can appreciate that it really does sound just one short step away from the funny farm. However, it's not as daft as it looks and it features a great deal in the 7 lbs in 7 Days programme.

Whenever you read anything about wheatgrass, nine times out of ten you will also hear the name Dr Anne Wigmore. Anne spent a considerable amount of her childhood learning about wheatgrass in Germany during the war. During this time, she and her grandmother were literally starving, but human nature being what it is, her survival instinct kicked in and they resorted to eating grass – or, more accurately, sucking the juice from it like many of us did when we were children. Later, she realized that during this period they never got sick and actually remained in very good health considering the apparent lack of nutrition on offer. Subsequently, Anne Wigmore became one of the pioneers of wheatgrass therapy research and nowadays there is extensive evidence of the health and healing powers of this plant. The application of wheatgrass therapy has been phenomenal and has even culminated in Anne founding the well-known Hippocrates Health Institutes.

Wheatgrass is grown from red wheat, a strain of wheat that is particularly nutritious and contains a variety of vitamins, minerals and trace elements. It is probably the most complete and beneficial nutritional drink available. One of the possible reasons for the effectiveness of wheatgrass might lie in its abundance of chlorophyll. Chlorophyll has a molecular structure resembling that of haemoglobin, the oxygen-carrying protein of red blood cells. Chlorophyll can be extracted from a majority of plants, but wheatgrass is one of the best sources as it has been found to contain over 100 key nutritional elements.

Wheatgrass is unlike the other fruits and vegetables on this plan, in that it can't simply be juiced in a centrifugal juicer, as this type of juicer cannot extract the juices from the grass. Likewise, it is not sufficient for us to eat the grass as we are not designed to digest the cellulose and would therefore only get a small percentage of the potential nutrients – and a painful stomach ache. This is probably a good thing as at this point your friends and loved ones might be tempted try to get you sectioned (confined to the nuthouse)!

There are a few different ways to obtain this amazing elixir (*see* **www.juicemaster.com** for further information). Essentially, you have three options: harvest and juice your own, get some 'ready-grown' wheatgrass, or use a good quality wheatgrass powder. The first option requires that you harvest and juice the wheatgrass yourself and for this you will need a separate masticating juice extractor. The second option is more convenient as it arrives at your house ready-grown. All you need to do is water it, cut some off and juice it. Then we have the ultra-convenient option of simply adding wheatgrass powder to your juice/smoothie.

JM's Wheatgrass Slammer©

There is also a brand-new way to get wheatgrass through a company in the UK that now delivers already-juiced wheatgrass to your door – frozen! It comes in handy 1oz shots and saves you the task of juicing. OK, frozen is never as good as fresh – but it's very close. You do not lose many nutrients when freezing foods, and more and more people are going for this option (see the link on my website). Personally, I still order fresh wheatgrass and juice it, but I'll often use the frozen option for convenience. I just love seeing wheatgrass in my house, and many people love teaching their kids how to grow it and juice it. The choice, as they say, is yours.

COWS EAT IT
DOPES SMOKE IT
THE *ENLIGHTENED* DRINK IT!

In my quest to Juice the World a few Juice Master Juice 'n' Smoothie bars have opened around the world. As I write, we have one in Ireland, one in Scotland, two in Dubai and one soon to open in Canada. If you visit one, you'll be able to get yourself a Juice Master Wheatgrass Slammer. If you wish to recreate the experience at home, here's a tip. Juice some fresh wheatgrass and put in a 1-oz shot cup. Put a little bit of rock salt on the back of your hand and have an orange quarter ready to bite into. Lick the salt, slam the wheatgrass and bite the orange. The taste of freshly-made wheatgrass juice isn't for everyone, but if you have it like a slammer, it's good to go on the taste front.

Ready-Grown or Grow Your Own

If you are going to juice fresh, then you can buy a tray of ready-grown wheatgrass, have some ready-cut wheatgrass sent to you or get a grow-your-own kit. The ready-grown trays are excellent and simply need watering. The ready-cut option is even easier –

it comes to your door already grown and cut, and will last 7 days. However, you might prefer the challenge and gratification of actually growing and tending your very own crop.

If you choose to do this, please bear in mind that the crop takes between 7 and 10 days before it is ready to be harvested, so to maintain momentum and get started as soon as possible with the 7 lbs in 7 Days programme it is probably best to use one of the alternative wheatgrass sources. If growing your own is for you, then I urge you to start cultivating some wheatgrass right now so you are fully prepared for Phases 2 and 3.

Wheatgrass Powder

You can buy 100% freeze-dried wheatgrass juice which, depending on how you look at it, takes away the hassle or the pleasure of growing, harvesting and juicing. If you are concerned about the quality, you won't be losing a great deal. Some experts say that wheatgrass powder 'preserves all the nutrients and enzymes for everyday vitality and well-being'. Using the powder is certainly easier and it also means that you don't need to buy a masticating juicer.

Psyllium Husks

Pronounced 'silly-um', these husks are far from silly. They contain a high level of soluble dietary fibre and because of this they are commonly prescribed for the treatment of constipation, diarrhoea and IBS. Psyllium is suitable for vegetarians, and it is not related to wheat so it does not contain gluten, yeast, dairy, sugar, salt or artificial colours and preservatives. When soaked in water, the husks swell into a gelatinous mass and maintain a high water content in the bowel. Once in the intestine they form a soft bulky mass that passes through the colon more smoothly and easily. All this is good news if you are either blocked up or finding it a little too easy to go! I recommend you add a heaped teaspoon of psyllium husks to one of your daily juices (preferably the early morning one), just to keep everything moving as nature intended!

This bulking agent does its job regardless of whether it's inside your body or simply incorporated into a juice waiting to be drunk. As a word of warning, please *do drink the juice as soon as it is made or put it straight into a sealed flask.* I found out to my cost just how efficient this bulking agent can be. After leaving my beautifully prepared juice for just half an hour I soon discovered it would be easier to eat it with a spoon than attempt to drink it!

The addition of psyllium husks to this plan is especially useful for helping to eliminate toxins, chemicals and waste products from the body. Once in the intestines, the psyllium traps and removes toxins, which might otherwise accumulate and back up into the body, causing symptoms such as headaches, loss of energy and fatigue. Another key attribute of psyllium is its potential to help with weight loss, due to its ability to make one feel full in the stomach. Medical studies have also shown that psyllium husks help to lower cholesterol levels, and therefore help protect against the risk of heart disease as well as help to balance blood sugar levels in people with diabetes.

Q & A

NOTE: This is a *must*-read part of the programme. You should read this before starting the programme.

Q: *I don't have a juicer. Can I do the programme if I just have a blender?*

A: NO, NO, NO – this is a juice programme and in order to make fresh juice you need a juicer extractor *and* a blender.

Q: *So what's the difference between a juicer and a blender?*

A: A juicer extracts the juice from the fibres of the fruits and vegetables whereas a blender simply 'chops' the *whole* fruit/veg fibre into a sort of 'mush'. I once went on Chiltern Radio's breakfast show simply because one of the presenters made the complete Turbo-Charge Smoothie

recipe in a blender only. The recipe relies on juicing many
of the ingredients and blending others. By simply blending
the lot she ended up with an awful mush of vegetables.

Q: *I own a blender. Do I need a smoothie maker as well?*

A: NO! One of the biggest marketing cons of the century
has to be that of the smoothie maker. Blenders *are*
smoothie makers! It's like someone selling a normal
saucepan and then calling it an 'egg boiling pan'. *All*
saucepans boil eggs and *all* blenders can make smoothies.
The only difference is that there is a tap on the front ...
genius! Whenever you see the words 'smoothie maker' or
'blender' you can rest assure they are one and the same
thing.

Q: *Do I have to do Phases 2 and 3 or is the 7-Day thing
enough?*

A: It is extremely important that even if you do choose to
skip the principles of the Phase 2 Turbo-Charge and Phase
3 Juicy Lifestyle plans you ease yourself into whole foods
during the two days immediately after the 7-Day plan,
effectively days 8 and 9. As was shown on the British TV
show *Celebrity Detox*, the body needs time to adjust in order
to go from pure natural juices to food, as the food can be
treated as a foreign invader and 'block' you up. When you
end a juice-only plan make sure you continue to have juice
for breakfast and lunch and a light evening meal on days 8

and 9 and then a juice for breakfast, a salad lunch and
evening meal on day 10. If you then wish to skip juicing
and go back to what you always ate and drank before you
started then that's your call. Personally, I think you'd be
mad and by going on Phases 2 and 3 you will ensure that
the weight you have lost and the health you have gained
will remain. If you choose the Phase 2 option of reading
the Turbo-Charge book on the day specified and starting
the Turbo-Charge programme immediately after the 7-day
plan, you will find you have both the physical and mental
tools required to take you to the next level.

Q: *Do I have to have a juice every three hours?*

A: No, you don't. The reason why the programme
suggests a juice every three hours is to prevent any dips in
sugar levels which can lead to a 'GIVE ME SOME FOOD
NOW!' response. When testing this programme on several
people, and through my own personal experience, it
appears that you don't have to have a juice every three
hours. When I first did the programme I had four juices the
first day, three the next and only two juices on the third
day. This was because on the evening of day 3 I just didn't
feel hungry. I felt a little tired and remember having a
lovely hot bath, reading a little and then lying on the bed
in that 'just out of a hot bath' haze listening to some
wonderful music, drinking some water and drifting off to
sleep. On day 4 I had a big meeting which took me away
from my house from 8 a.m. until 11 p.m. I had to improvise

and had three flasks of juice with me. I only ended up drinking about a litre and a half of the juice, together with drinking plenty of water. However, on day 5 I felt genuinely hungry and I had all five juices. Whatever happens you want to make sure you have some made up just in case you get hungry, to prevent any chance of bingeing.

Q: *Do I have to keep exactly to the juices suggested on each day or can I make my own combo?*

A: The juices and smoothies aren't just thrown together and the order has been carefully thought out. However, please feel free to be flexible when it comes to making them. Sometimes you can't get hold of certain produce, or you may not feel like a particular juice/smoothie. You may also particularly like a certain smoothie and want to keep to that. I know some people who LOVED the Super, Detox and Turbo Express so much that that's all they had. Changing recipes is fine as long as you stick to a couple of basic rules.

➤ Always use apple, pineapple or carrot or a combination of these as a base to your veggie juices.
➤ Make sure you always add a teaspoon of psyllium husk powder for a natural source of dietary fibre – so you don't get stuck!
➤ Add a small amount of spirulina, wheatgrass powder and friendly bacteria to your juices/smoothies for added super-nutrients.

This doesn't mean you need to add these supplements for every juice, but you do need to make sure that at least two have the above.

Q: *What should I do when eating out on the programme?*

A: Quite simply, DON'T! There is no eating on this programme, but you are welcome to take your flask! I know that sounds ridiculous, but when I did this for the first time I had meetings, lunches, dinners and so on to contend with. I know from personal experience that nothing can prevent you from following this programme to the letter if you really want to – except you, that is.

Q: *Can I eat fruit or veg if I don't feel like juicing it?*

A: Yes and No! Firstly, this is a 'juice only' programme and that means if you are going to do it to the letter you won't be using your teeth for a week. Having said that, if it's a case of *'Unless I eat something, ANYTHING – NOW! – I'm going to forget the whole thing and eat a horse,'* then at least make sure you eat something good. The best suggestion is to eat foods with an extremely high water content, like fruits and vegetables. The best choice is melon. I had to go out for a business dinner when I was doing the programme and I ordered a piece of melon – it tasted amazing. If you hit a particular evening and you feel that for whatever reason you really cannot face juice and want to get your teeth into something other than fruit, have a large well-prepared avocado salad.

Q: *Can I drink anything else other than freshly made juice on the programme?*

A: Yes. You will see that in the programme you are encouraged to drink at least two litres of water a day and drink some hot water and lemon on waking and natural fennel tea at night. However, you are most welcome to have mint tea or other herbal teas if you fancy.

Q: *Can I drink bottled juices/smoothies while on the programme if I don't have the time to juice fresh?*

A: If push really comes to shove then yes, but only in absolute emergencies. The reality is that if you are fully prepared there are very few situations where you cannot get a fresh juice or make a fresh juice. If someone offered you a million pounds to make sure you had a fresh juice every time – trust me you'd do whatever it took. However, I'm also aware that unexpected 'stuff' can come up in life and best intentions can often go out of the window. With that in mind here are my suggestions for juices when out and about.

1 **Direct from a juice bar.** If you have a juice bar near you then ask them to make up the exact juice you want and make sure you can see them making it. Many juice bars have 'ready-made' juices in coolers – these are almost always not freshly extracted juices. You are the paying

customer and even if you have to pay more – get the real thing. If by the time you read this the **Juice Master®** chain of juice bars is up and running around the country, then you can be sure we will make you any juice or smoothie you like. If you are in a regular juice bar and they cannot make the exact juice you want, then just make up a juice from their menu of fruit and veggie choices. Many juice bars will not have the likes of cucumber, spinach, courgette and so on, but they nearly always have carrot, apple, ginger and lemon – so you can ask for the Lemon/Ginger Zinger (*see* page 158). Most juice bars now do shots of wheatgrass, so have one of those either in your juice or as a chaser.

2 **A 'good' bottled juice.** ALL juices that are in bottle form on shelves in supermarkets and the like have been pasteurized. This process lowers the vitamin and mineral content and destroys the enzyme activity – the life force contained within the plant. Also, it is almost impossible to get a good 'veggie' bottled juice and most are fruit based. I would suggest that if you are going to 'hit the bottle' then you should go for 100% pure juices not made from concentrate. However, remember these have also been pasteurized.

Q: *I smoke. Do I need to stop smoking in order to have success on the programme?*

A: That depends on what your idea of success is. Clearly it would always be better to stop smoking whether you are doing this programme or not, but since I used to smoke 40–60 cigarettes a day myself I'm fully aware that without the right knowledge and guidance stopping smoking can be a frightening prospect.

If you are doing this programme to lose weight then whether you are smoking or not will not make a difference. If you want to lose weight *and* get healthy then clearly stopping would be good – but you know that already. But if you feel that you cannot stop smoking then I would advise that you still do the programme. You will always be healthier than you are now and with the tremendous amount of antioxidants going into your system throughout the week, it will do wonders to counter the effect of the **4,000 chemicals** found in your average cigarette.

People who smoke often ask, 'If I stop smoking will I gain weight?' Stopping smoking does not make you fat – FOOD makes you fat – or TOO MUCH FOOD, to be more accurate. If you stop smoking and do this programme you have the best of both worlds. You won't get fat and you will have cleaned your body of all the nicotine within just three days. YES, it doesn't matter how long you have been smoking or what your intake is, it takes just three days for your system to be clear of nicotine – though I'm afraid the tarry residue is another matter entirely. However, it's not your system that is addicted to nicotine; it's primarily your mind. If you need help to stop smoking easily and painlessly go to **www.juicemaster.com** and get hold of the 'Stop Smoking in 2 Hours' double CD programme. Imagine getting healthy, losing more than 7 lbs and stopping smoking all in a week. What we *can* do is incredible, what we are *willing* to do is often anything but – it's your call.

Q: *If I have a wheat intolerance can I still have wheatgrass juice?*

A: Yes. Having had a major and now slight intolerance to wheat this was one of the first questions I asked. Wheatgrass is the young grass stage of wheat grain plants, taken just after sprouting. This means that at this stage it is a leafy plant and not a grain and so is completely gluten free. When people have a wheat intolerance it usually means they have an intolerance to the gluten in the wheat grains.

Q: *I am constipated. When can I expect to go again?*

A: When people either embark on this plan or come on a juice retreat, around 20% of them experience a 'blockage', so to speak. This is nothing to worry about and all will soon be moving with the Phase 2 Turbo-Charge and Phase 3 Juicy Lifestyle plans. However, in order to address this problem I have added some whole apple to some recipes that is blended into the juice. This combination gives plenty of soluble and insoluble fibre, which should keep things moving. If you do stay 'stuck' then eat some prunes, have some prune juice or see your GP to see if there's anything else that could be wrong.

Q: *I have the opposite problem ... I can't stop going. Can you help?*

A: Firstly, it's nothing to worry about, and secondly, see it as a free colonic! This is often a very good sign – it's the body chucking out the built-up rubbish. If, however, your 'waste' is simply coming out too fast, then here's a tip. Add more of the psyllium husks to your juices. When this happens it's often because people haven't bothered to add any psyllium husks at all. Please remember, everything is here for a reason.

Q: *My poo is sometimes red. Should I worry?*

A: Your poo may well be red for one of two reasons. The first is the most common – **raw beetroot**. If you have a juice containing raw beetroot the chances are that at some point soon after traces of the strong red pigment will be found in your 'waste'. This is nothing whatsoever to worry about and if you continue to have beet in your juices then the colour will soon return to normal.

The second reason could be you that you actually have blood in your poo. If you have then the chances are you have haemorrhoids. If this is the case it is unlikely to be anything to worry about. It means you have 'strained' too hard and burst a small blood vessel in that area. This usually repairs in a day or two. If it continues, ALWAYS go to your GP and get it checked.

Q: *I've done 5 days. Is that enough?*

A: No. This is a *7-day* programme. It's only 7 days and anyone can do anything for 7 days – *if* they are committed to it. If you really feel that the whole 7 days will take you 'over the edge' and would mean you getting very deprived to the point of having the ultimate 'SOD IT' mood and start bingeing on rubbish, then, yes, 5 days is enough. What I would strongly suggest is that you still have a juice for breakfast, a juice, smoothie, salad or some fruit for lunch and an evening meal that consists of either organic chicken with wholegrain rice, some steamed veggies or a large mixed salad.

Q: *I have just finished the programme and I haven't lost 7 lbs. Can you explain this?*

A: The ideal time to weigh yourself is the night before you start the programme and then the morning of day 8, making sure you have exactly the same clothes on. If you have done this and haven't lost 7 lbs – as happens in some cases – the result will usually appear one, two or three days after you finish the 7-day programme. If you haven't lost the weight by then, the chances are that you weren't very overweight to start with and your body doesn't want to drop to an unhealthy weight. (It is remotely possible that you may be one of the *very* few people in the world with a genuine thyroid problem that could prevent weight loss. If you were overweight to start with, have followed the programme rigorously, and have still not lost any weight, then you should get yourself checked over by a doctor to be on the safe side.)

Q: *Can I drink any tea, coffee or alcohol on the programme?*

A: What do you think?

Q: *Can I make a big batch and store it for a few days to save having to make it all the time?*

A: You should always make juice fresh whenever you can – 'fresh is best', as they say. The next best thing is to make some, add a bit of lemon or lime juice and seal it *immediately*, then put it in the fridge and drink it within the next eight hours. Remember, though, that with every hour that passes you lose more and more nutrients, so drink it as soon as you can. Having said that, if you still have some in a flask after 12–14 hours, don't throw it away; it will still have plenty of vitamins, minerals, fats, carbohydrates and some amino acids. But fresh is best whenever you can.

Q: *I 'm getting headaches and I have no energy, I feel so tired and it's only day 2!*

A: When the body is detoxing, depending on just how 'toxic' the person was to start with, it is quite common to experience headaches and *initial* energy loss. You need to understand that you were falsely stimulating your body and covering up what was really going on. What you are experiencing is your 'true' level of health (sorry to scare you!). After 3 days the headaches should subside and after 3–4 days you should start to get a great deal more energy. It is important that if you feel like this you do the *light* exercises part of the programme as movement gives you energy; remember, total rigidity = death! To feel alive you have to move.

Q: *I feel sick and am getting stomach aches. Is this normal and what should I do?*

A: No, this is not normal: headaches – yes; tiredness – yes; nausea – no! Nausea can happen to some people going on juice plans for the first time but it shouldn't last longer than a day while your system adjusts to the juices. You may be drinking them too fast; always 'chew' your juice – make sure you keep it in the mouth and allow the powerful enzymes in your saliva to make good contact with the juice. You may be making the recipes wrong and perhaps drinking too many 'neat' green juices. Green juices, with the exception of celery and cucumber, should always be mixed with other juices such as carrot, apple and pineapple. If you are making the juices correctly, are drinking them slowly, and you are still feeling nausea after day 1 – come off the plan IMMEDIATELY and see your GP.

Q: *I'm allergic to _____ . What shall I do?*

A: I remember once being on the shopping channel QVC and a lady called and said, 'I have your book [not this one] and a juicer and I love my new juicy life. However, I'm allergic to strawberries and onions. What should I do?' Unfortunately, I'm not very good at hiding my disbelief at certain questions – even on live TV. My reply was, 'Go on, have a wild stab in the dark. What do you think you should do? Don't have them!' It was a silly question as she wasn't on a programme that advised either strawberry juice or onion juice. I often encounter people who are allergic to some of the fruit and veg that are in this programme and if that's the case then you just need to use your imagination. If you are allergic to apples then use pineapple instead; if allergic to carrots use apples. The key is to know that in order to make any of the veggie-based juices taste OK, the base should be made up of either carrot, apple or pineapple. If you are allergic to all three of these, then you are in trouble on this programme. Having said that, I have yet to find anyone who is allergic to *all three* of these ingredients. Please also bear in mind that just because you have a mild reaction to a particular fruit or veg when you eat it, it doesn't always mean that the same applies when you have it juiced.

Q: *I lost more than 7 lbs. Should I worry?*

A: Nope! If you've lost more than 7 lbs on this plan then the chances are you needed to lose it anyway. I know many people who have lost more and one who even lost 14 lbs – it all depends on the person, to what degree they did the programme, how much exercise they took and how big they were to start with. Just make sure you do the Phase 2 Turbo-Charge plan so you introduce food back into you diet *correctly*. You will not necessarily have lost 7 lbs of fat – in all likelihood you won't have – but a combination of 7 lbs of excess fat, water *and* other stuff that you needed to get rid of. The only time losing more weight is bad is if you were already thin and have got even thinner doing this. The idea is to get slim, not 'thin'. The good news is that even if this has happened, you have lost too much and are looking as if you are about to snap – so to speak – as long as you complete Phase 2 and the Phase 3 Juicy Lifestyle plan your body should return to a normal weight.

Q: *It's a pain having to clean the machine after every use. Is there a way around this?*

A: The day they invent a self-cleaning juicer is the day when everyone in the country will start juicing. Cleaning the machine can be a pain at times (some machines are more of a pain than others) but there is a method where you simply clean the machine once or twice a day. When making a juice, make sure you place a bag into the 'pulp' compartment (assuming your machine has a separate one – all good ones do) so that you can simply take out the bag after using the machine. Then run the machine and pour a little warm water into it. You can then leave the machine for a couple of hours and all should be fine. Having said that, it is ALWAYS BETTER to clean the machine immediately after using it (*see* 'Your 10 Steps to Quick and Easy Juicing', page 202). For those who really, really can't get into the whole juicing and cleaning, I have developed the 7lbs in 7 Days Delivery System. This is where you simply call a number and get all your juices and smoothies delivered to your home or office every day. No shopping, no cleaning, no juicing and no hassle. Please see website to see if this service is available where you are.

Q: *Can I do this programme if I'm pregnant?*

A: That's not straightforward to answer. I don't know anything about you and I wouldn't want you to jump into this programme and then find something is wrong. As always, when in doubt consult your GP first. Having said this, I can't see how it could possibly be harmful – I would have thought that if you were pregnant you would require more avocado and larger portions – but please check.

Q: *Is this programme suitable for children?*

A: Yes, but not very young children, only for those aged 10 years or more. As with any dietary programme, do ask your GP first, as he or she knows your child's medical history.

Q: *I want to come on one of your 7-day Intimate Juice Retreats. Where do I get info on them?*

A: All information regarding our retreats can be found on the website (**www.juicemaster.com**) or you can speak to a real-life person on the juicy hotline (0845 130 2829 – local call anywhere in the UK). On a retreat, the juice detox experience will usually be much easier and more enjoyable and successful than when you do it yourself and are trying to fit it in around your work, home and social life. The reason for this is twofold:

1 You are away from it all and are having your juices made for you.
2 You are up a mountain with very few pollutants. And, as well as being in an extremely positive environment, you will have the opportunity to do yoga (aimed at all levels), mini-rebounding (the best form of exercise in world – *so say NASA*), great walks, good-quality water and freshly grown organic wheatgrass. The juicy team will tell you more when you call.

Q: *How often should I go on the programme?*

A: Once a season. Even if all else went pear-shaped on the health and fitness front, you will know that at the start of every three months you do at least the 7-day programme. Ideally you would do the 7 lbs in 7 Days Super Juice Diet, immediately followed by the Phase 2 Turbo-Charge programme. I cannot emphasize enough just how powerful the combination of these two programmes is. It is also an excellent idea to read the Turbo Book (or listen to the Turbo CD) while you are on the 7 lbs in 7 Days programme. This will once again re-inspire you, put you into the right way of thinking and make the process not only easy but enjoyable. If you are not familiar with the Turbo book or don't fancy it, then do the whole of this programme – Phases 1, 2 and 3 of the 7 lbs in 7 Days programme.

Q: *I thought I'd learn a lot more about juicing in this book. Is there any reason why there isn't more information about what juices are for what illnesses and so on?*

A: Yes. Juicing is such a complex subject and if I had included all of the information on every disease and what juices can help and so on, the book would have been three times the size. For more information on juicing, get hold of *The Juice Master's Keeping it Simple.*

Q: *Where can I get the 7 lbs in 7 Days Super Juice Pack? Do I really need it?*

A: From the website (**www.juicemaster.com**) or by calling the juicy hotline (0845 130 2829). The question of whether you really need the 7-day pack is one which only you can answer. Personally, I would get the pack, or at least the CD and DVD if nothing else, as I'm more of an audiovisual person than a devotee of the written word – which might seem weird since I write books. I also like to have some encouragement and a degree of support along the way, and once you are in the right frame of mind you don't need support and the rest is pretty easy. The pack also contains this book so you may wish to just buy the CD and DVD separately.

Q: *When and where are your 7lbs in 7 Days Detox Retreats?*

A: At the time of writing they are in southern Turkey. I have two venues. The main 7lbs in 7 Days Retreat home is high in the mountains with breathtaking views and a sunset to die for. The second retreat venue is my main event venue and is set in one of the most unique boutique hotels on earth. We even have our own private Island where we rebound until morning sunrise! On the back page are a small sample of the letters and e-mails from the retreats. Hope to meet you there in person one day soon.

Juice Master Info

For information on Juice Master books, CDs, DVDs, forthcoming seminars, juice-bar opportunities plus anything else you need to know about our juicy world:

Call the Juice Master Hotline: 08451 30 28 29 (this is a *local call* charge from anywhere in the UK)
Website: www.juicemaster.com
E-mail: info@juicemaster.com

The Juice Master's Mind and Body Detox Retreats

An amazing experience. You spend a week in a beautiful European costal destination, drinking only the finest-quality freshly extracted juices, doing yoga, meditation, meeting new people and attending seminars designed to change the way you think about what you feed yourself. These are only held a few times a year and Jason is usually at each event, but places go fast. For more info, see our website or speak to one of the juicy team.

> 'It's so amazing what can happen in just one week. It is much more than just about weight loss, I feel like I faced all my angels and demons and am just ready for the world. Hope you are all feeling on top of the world too.'
> **Tosh, 13th August 2009**

NOTE: The money off vouchers are not in conjunction with any other offer.

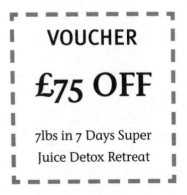

VOUCHER	VOUCHER
£75 OFF	**£75 OFF**
7lbs in 7 Days Super Juice Detox Retreat	One Week *Ultimate* Mind and Body Juice Retreat

What People Say About the 7lbs in 7 Days Retreat ...

'I'm 12lbs lighter and feel a hundred times better than when I arrived in Turkey. Mum lost 7lbs and is thrilled ... I'm beginning to feel how I have wanted to feel for a long time, and I certainly can't remember the last time I felt so positive and so relaxed ... thank you so much for your warmth and kindness and for helping me to feel the way I do now – free, happy and full of love and life.'
Kathryn

'Holy S**T! ... Ok, just got back home from retreat and got on the scales next morning. I had to get off and on again as I thought the scale was broken. Got back on and my jaw dropped ... I lost 15lbs! 15LBS! ... in one week!! WOW. I felt great before I left the retreat but now I am just buzzing. I've been doing yoga, bouncing and running every morning since I got back and loving it. Bring it on!'
Gary

'I loved the week with you wish I was still there. I've lost 10lb, and have kept it off ...!! So grateful to you, feel great, husband thinks I've lost the plot leaping out of bed everyday at 6.30!!! Have booked for next year, second shop will be open by then ... Good luck with everything, I'm spreading the word.'
Claire A.